PRESERVING THE ETCHINGS OF THE MIND

AGING, DEMENTIA, AND HEARING LOSS

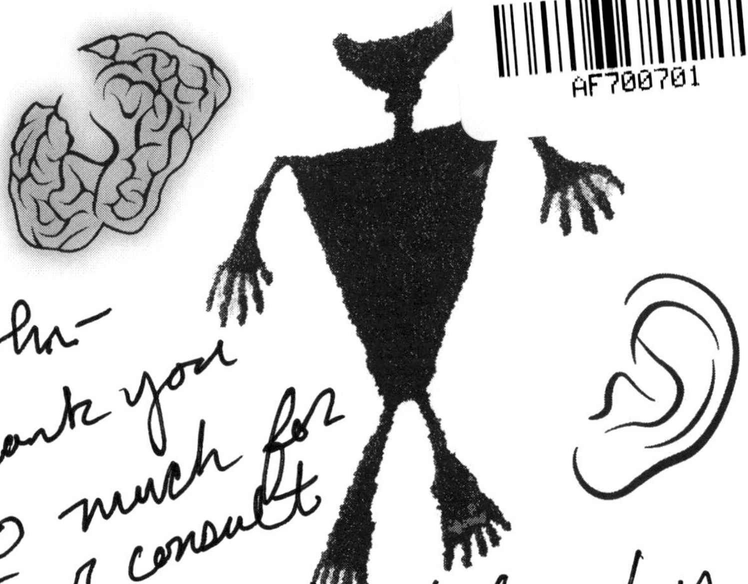

DR. JAIME A.B. WILSON

ILLUSTRATIONS BY GREY KAMPS
AND ANN WILSON

John – Thank you so much for your consult & expertise today! You are indispensible in our hearing loss world! Jaime Wilson 06/26/24

First Edition, 2023

Published by Savory Words Publishing
www.savorywords.com

978-1-7377117-7-3
Printed in the United States of America

WHAT OTHERS SAY ABOUT THIS BOOK

This book covers such important and, in ways, novel territory. Dr. Wilson provides essential information for individuals with hearing loss to keep the brain healthy, vital, and engaged. The primary auditory pathways and auditory association cortical areas comprise a substantial part of the brain. *Etchings of the Mind* elaborates on how to keep these critical neural systems active and adaptive as the brain ages.

Dr. Erin D. Bigler, Ph.D., ABPP
Board-certified Neuropsychologist
Emeritus Professor and Director, MRI Research Laboratory
Brigham Young University

This book will help empower individuals with hearing loss to proactively address their needs to manage their potential risks for cognitive decline. By arming them with this valuable information, they can engage their healthcare providers and healthcare systems meaningfully and ensure that they are not marginalized or ignored with respect to their healthcare needs.

Dr. Michael M. McKee, MD, MPH
Board-certified Family Medicine Physician
Deaf Health Clinic at Dexter Health Center
University of Michigan Medical School

In *Preserving the Etchings of the Mind,* Dr. Wilson delivers an exceptional review of the dementia risk factors, including hearing loss. He addresses the all-important issue of medical conditions that, once addressed, resolves the underlying dementia-like condition. Dr. Wilson also provides tools, evidence-based insights, and pharmacological options for reducing the risk of cognitive decline and leading healthier lives today.

Dr. David S. Shearer, Ph.D., MSCP, ABMP
Board-certified Prescribing Medical Psychologist
Madigan Army Medical Center (MAMC)
Director of Behavioral Sciences, Family Medicine Residency

This book helps clarify the hearing loss and dementia connection while also providing current trends in behavioral and pharmacological options to improve our odds of staying mentally sharp. The book is well-written and flows very nicely, providing a background on dementia. Dr. Wilson's style of writing is informative and relaxed, with good examples that are easily relatable and will keep the reader's interest. He does not burden the reader with jargon; instead, he provides a logical connection between dementia and hearing loss. I highly recommend this book.

Dr. Randall L. Tackett, Ph.D.
Professor of Clinical and Administrative Pharmacy
Associate Department Head
College of Pharmacy, University of Georgia

Dr. Wilson's book is a solid introduction to dementia. It keeps in perspective the things we can do to reduce the risk of cognitive decline and brings special attention to the relationship between hearing loss and dementia. His writing style is friendly and relatable, with a light, easily understandable approach to understanding dementia, its known risk factors, and lifestyle changes that may mitigate the onset and progression of dementia. The book is full of useful contemporary information derived from the scientific literature, presented in understandable terms that will have wide appeal.

Dr. Munro Cullum, Ph.D., ABPP
Board-certified Neuropsychologist
Professor of Psychiatry, Neurology,
and Neurological Surgery
Scientific Director, Texas Alzheimer's Research
and Care Consortium
University of Texas Southwestern Medical Center

Dr. Wilson has a way of helping us see and hear things in new ways. In this excellent, accessible, and fun book, he helps illuminate the mystery of the hearing loss-dementia connection and provides practical advice on reducing the risk of cognitive decline.

Dr. Glenn E. Smith, Ph.D., ABPP
Board-certified Neuropsychologist
Director of the Florida Alzheimer's Disease Research Center
University of Florida Faculty Member

Our understanding of the relationship between hearing loss, aging, and dementia has greatly expanded in recent decades. In this book, Dr. Wilson provides an easy-to-read, accessible, and thorough summary of these important topics, along with proactive solutions and recommendations as we advance in age.

Dr. Samuel R. Atcherson, Ph.D., FNAP
Professor of Audiology and Otolaryngology—
Head and Neck Surgery
University of Arkansas for Medical Sciences

Dr. Wilson has provided a valuable addition to the literature on an enormous topic that has repercussions for many who experience hearing loss. This is a well-researched and actionable guide for limiting the risk factors associated with dementia. It is a welcome regimen to counter the sense of hopelessness many feel when facing age-related cognitive decline.

Dr. Christopher J. Moreland, MD, MPH
Board-certified Internist Physician
Associate Professor, Department of Internal Medicine and
Associate Program Director, Internal Medicine Residency
Dell Medical School, University of Texas at Austin

This is a clear account of how hearing loss functions as a risk factor for dementia. Dr. Wilson draws on both his personal experience as a Deaf person as well as his extensive knowledge of the scientific literature. The result is a book that not only informs about how bad dementia can get but also what one can do to protect one's brain health. This book is readily accessible to both the lay public and early career professionals. It should be in the library of anybody who works with patients who are Deaf or have late-onset hearing loss.

Dr. Jacobs Donders, Ph.D., ABPP
Board-certified Neuropsychologist
Mary Free Bed Rehabilitation Hospital

In *Preserving the Etchings of the Mind*, Dr. Wilson presents a concise, easy-to-understand review of the basic dementing conditions. The primary value of Dr. Wilson's book may be its inclusion of chapters on the relationship between hearing loss and dementia, an area that has been almost entirely excluded in other books on dementia. Given his own hearing loss, Dr. Wilson concisely describes the reasons individuals with hearing loss may experience dementia and, more importantly, strategies to decrease this likelihood. This book is likely to be a standard for those who work with the hearing loss population.

Dr. Brick Johnstone, Ph.D., ABPP
Board-certified Neuropsychologist
Director, Brain Injury Research Shepherd Center

Etchings of the Mind provides guidance on keeping the brain vital and active, thereby giving us the best tools to maximize quality of life during our later years. Dr. Wilson's book is an essential read for individuals with hearing loss from all walks of life and a useful tool for clinicians as well—he weaves together clinical and practical information seamlessly.

Dr. Jennifer L. Reesman, Ph.D., ABPP
Board-certified Neuropsychologist
Director of Training and Assessments
The Chesapeake Center

Dr. Wilson's enthusiasm in spreading awareness of the connections between dementia and hearing loss is palpable throughout this highly accessible book. *Etchings of the Mind* is a must-read for individuals and those who have loved ones with hearing loss.

Dr. Allen E. Thornton, Ph.D., ABPP
Board-certified Neuropsychologist
Professor of Human Neuropsychology Laboratory
Simon Fraser University

Dr. Wilson has written a highly engaging and readable book about the association between hearing loss and dementia. He gives practical information without fearmongering and instills a sense of confidence and optimism about the role lifestyle can play in reducing dementia risk. Wonderful book!

Dr. Suzanne Penna, Ph.D., ABPP-CN
Board-certified Neuropsychologist
Associate Professor and Director of the Division of Rehabilitation Neuropsychology
Emory University School of Medicine

I recognize the importance of providing education for youth who may become the next generation of caretakers for their loved ones experiencing cognitive decline. It is never too early for family members to learn about dementia and its associated risk factors, especially that of hearing loss. This book presents a wealth of information that may alleviate many of the common fears among individuals and families with loved ones who experience cognitive decline. Additionally, readers of all ages may benefit from this discussion of lifestyle choices that can reduce the risk of dementia.

Dr. Alice Ann Holland, Ph.D., ABPP
Board-certified Pediatric Neuropsychologist
Children's Medical Center Dallas

Dr. Wilson is at the forefront of the latest research on hearing and brain health. It is with great confidence that I recommend him and this book to assist with behavioral and pharmacological interventions for maximizing brain health.

Dr. Brandon Henscheid, Psy.D., MSCP
Prescribing Medical Psychologist
Wilson Clinical Services, PLLC

This book provides an excellent update on the most common types of brain disorders underlying dementia and also takes a deep dive into understanding the relationship between hearing loss and dementia. This is a common yet not often discussed topic within dementia science. This book also provides up-to-date recommendations on pharmaceutical as well as behavior approaches in maintaining optimal cognitive functioning. A practical book for both the layperson and professional.

Dr. Ryan Ernst, Psy.D., MSCP, ABN
Prescribing Medical Psychologist and
Board-certified Neuropsychologist
Director of Training in Psychopharmacology,
Department of Pharmacy and Health Sciences
Drake University

This book is an excellent primer on the common types of dementia, as well as a behind-the-scenes look at the dementia risk factors associated with hearing loss. Both late-onset and early-onset hearing loss are examined, including those individuals belonging to the Deaf ASL-using community. The recommendations included in this book for protecting the brain are essential reading for consumers wishing to take active steps toward the preservation of their long-term brain health.

Dr. Nathan Glassman, Ph.D., ABN, ABPP
Board-certified Neuropsychologist and
Clinical Psychologist (Retired)

Dr. Wilson is our guide into the world of dementia. Like the true educator he is, he explains the different causes in a way that is a cut above layman's terms. As a result, even readers who may be familiar with some terms used by medical professionals will better understand their meanings and implications. Most importantly, Dr.

Wilson highlights an often-overlooked risk factor for dementia—hearing loss.

I hope readers will appreciate factors that can accompany hearing loss, such as social isolation and stressed cognitive resources, and take steps to mitigate these. Dr. Wilson notes that we recall better when we have fun while learning, and, like the best guides, he sprinkles amusing quotes and anecdotes along the way to keep us engaged. I certainly enjoyed this journey and expect you will too.

Dr. Kathleen Fuchs, Ph.D., ABPP
Board-certified Neuropsychologist
Director of Postdoctoral Training
University of Virginia Department of Neurology and Memory and Aging Care Clinic

As a colleague with hearing loss, Dr. Wilson recognizes the urgency for practical and easy-to-read recommendations to keep the mind as healthy as possible. This book is chock full of beneficial advice for keeping fit on a physical and psychological level. We would all benefit from following even half the book's recommendations.

Dr. Danielle M. Previ, Ph.D.
Licensed Clinical Psychologist
Kennedy Krieger Institute

Dr. Wilson does an excellent job simplifying complex and important research into a practical guide for dementia prevention. His passion and knowledge provide insight into the connection between hearing loss and dementia.

Dr. Glen Getz, Ph.D., ABN
Board-certified Neuropsychologist
Neuropsychology Specialty Care

In a landscape that has needed an authoritative book to connect brain health and hearing, *Preserving the Etchings of the Mind* masterfully brings together decades of research and clinical experience in a very readable and relatable format. This book is a must-have for anyone interested in learning about ways to protect and preserve our brains.

Dr. Farzin Irani, Ph.D., ABPP
Board-certified Neuropsychologist
AAA Neuropsychology

This book is scientifically based, delightfully readable, and full of up-to-date information. Not only will you learn about different types of dementias and risk factors but also about treatments, including lifestyle changes and current pharmacotherapy. I know of no other book on dementia that is as informative and as easy to read. Dr. Wilson encourages readers that it is never too late to start doing something about dementia and shows you where to start. And that, my friends, is worth its weight in gold.

Dr. Lynette Pujol, Ph.D., MSCP
Prescribing Medical Psychologist
Fairleigh Dickinson University Adjunct Professor
Society for Prescribing Psychology Research Council Chair

DEDICATION

This book is dedicated to all members of my darling family.

To my dear wife, Ann: true romance always has insider stuff. You are one of the greatest blessings in my life. I love you to an eight-turned-sideways.

To my precious children: you bring light and joy to each day of my life. No words can sufficiently describe how much I love each of you.

To my mom, Marlene. You taught me what it means to be a husband, dad, son, friend, and to love unconditionally. Thank you for raising me.

Thank you, Papa David, for caring for my mom and being who you are: a great man and stepdad.

To my dad, JAB. Not a day goes by without me thinking of you. I miss you. Until we meet again.

To my mother-in-law and father-in-law Sharrie and Jim: Thank you for being there more times than I can count. You both are angels in disguise.

To my Aunt Rachelle and Uncle Norman, thank you for your ongoing support and contagious enthusiasm for life.

And last but not least, this book is dedicated to the memory of my cousin Bernie Kaplan, who always encouraged me to write a book. Our intimate discussions over the Bernie and Mae salad in a Key West restaurant will be fondly remembered forever.

CONTENTS

PREFACE

It is no surprise that dementia is one of the biggest health obstacles to aging well. The well-respected medical journal, *The Lancet,* indicates that there are presently more than 50 million people living with dementia worldwide, with a forecasted increase to over a whopping 130 million people by 2050, Clearly, this is a healthcare phenomenon that deserves our care and attention. Bringing awareness to the general public regarding the hearing loss and dementia connection can help optimize strategies to protect against cognitive decline. *The Lancet* further notes that hearing loss is considered the most modifiable risk factor for dementia.

This book aims to spread awareness about the connection between hearing loss and dementia. Hearing loss is one of the most significant risk factors for dementia, accounting for 8% of all cases. These cases include individuals with late-onset hearing loss in middle age (ages 45-65) and those experiencing hearing loss from a young age (usually those who identify as culturally Deaf).

Several studies have shown that hearing loss appears to double the risk of dementia. As hearing loss worsens, the risk of dementia increases. Incident dementia increases across mild, moderate, and severe hearing loss levels, with severe hearing loss leading to five times the risk for dementia.

In Chapter 1, a common question is discussed regarding what constitutes "normal aging." This is differentiated from the four most common dementia types in Chapter 2. By increasing our awareness of common dementia conditions, we can be better prepared to seek timely interventions.

People with hearing loss can also minimize the risk of dementia by being aware of the known risk factors discussed in Chapter 3. We do have a lot of control over how well we age. Approximately 40% of dementias are thought to be preventable by addressing general risk factors.

Towards the end of this book (Chapters 4 and 5), we talk about proactive choices we can make to protect and preserve our brains. Lifestyle choices can go a long way toward minimizing the increased risk of dementia that hearing loss unfortunately presents. This is part of a powerful armamentarium we can use to our advantage in keeping dementia at bay.

In addition to increasing awareness of the dementia and hearing loss connection, I hope you will feel instilled with a sense of purpose, motivation, and joy in making the most out of a healthy lifestyle.

Here's to happiness and health for you and your loved ones!

FOREWORD

I started reading this book as a clinical psychologist, but then I found myself personally drawn to the topic. As a clinical psychologist, I have worked with colleagues to establish the clinical specialty of mental healthcare for deaf and hard of hearing people (what I prefer to call deaf mental health care).

I have produced six books on this developing discipline. I've written multiple peer-reviewed publications about how providers in deaf mental health care need to demonstrate 1) cultural and personal self-awareness about one's own multiple identities, including as deaf and hearing people, 2) a solid knowledge base related to diverse D/deaf people, deaf cultures and communities, 3) specialized communication and language skills, and 4) specialized skills in adapting best practices in mental health for diverse D/deaf people. I believe that practicing deaf mental health care well requires all of this.

Dr. Wilson's book makes a vital contribution to the deaf mental health care field, exploring the connection between hearing loss, deafness, and cognitive decline, and, importantly, doing so from a vantage point of respect for the deaf community. For instance, many deaf people who were raised without adequate sign language and who have not been able to communicate well with spoken language struggle to communicate even with their own families. This is all too common and tragic. Some of these people may never find a community of their own, missing out on the opportunity for life-affirming belonging in the deaf community. This lifelong communication, and social isolation, is profoundly disabling and now we know it also poses a risk for dementia.

Also at risk are hearing people who lose their hearing as they age but won't consider ways to remediate the problem, like using hearing aids. As their hearing declines, they may lose connection with their loved ones. Would knowing that this avoidable social isolation can contribute to cognitive decline persuade them to consider hearing aids and other adaptive technology?

Chapter 4, "Hearing Loss as a Risk Factor for Dementia," is an essential contribution to the deaf mental health care knowledge base. Dr. Wilson summarizes research showing how hearing loss is a risk factor for dementia, especially in cases of language deprivation in childhood. With over 40 years of work in this field, I did not fully appreciate this.

This connection between hearing loss and cognitive problems is a complex topic to discuss well because it may reinforce a medical-pathological, as opposed to a cultural, view of deaf people. Dr. Wilson, who is a Deaf, articulate ASL user, along with being an accomplished prescribing medical psychologist and board-certified neuropsychologist, sensitively describes both the medical and environmental contributions to cognitive decline in some deaf people. He is a highly credible source for an objective understanding of this problem.

Soon after I began the book, I realized, however, that the topic was personal to me. I am a 68-year-old hearing man who, like everyone I know of a certain age, worries about cognitive decline. There are two English sayings about aging that I think young people are frequently remiss in understanding. The first is commonly credited to George Bernard Shaw: youth is wasted on the young. When we are young, we don't always see all the possibilities before us, all the opportunities to seize, but when we are old, it's all too easy to look back and kick ourselves for not being more adventurous, more open to the world, even more generous of spirit. We often regret most not what we did but what we did not do or what we did not become. We say, "I wish I knew when I was young what I know now."

The second English saying is that "getting old ain't for wimps." When we are young, we may see our elders sharing stories of how their bodies are starting to fail them and think that this is a ridiculous topic to discuss. I certainly did. When we are old, we feel more vulnerable. We appreciate more deeply that our time is limited, and therefore each day, each moment is precious. We worry more about decline and loss and naturally want to check in with friends and family at a similar stage of life.

For most elderly people I know, cognitive decline is a chief source of worry, often relieved through humor. I jokingly reassure myself and them constantly by saying, "Well, we may misplace our keys more, but at least we still know what the keys are for," or "I haven't yet left the keys in the refrigerator." We console ourselves by talking about "senior moments." We all know what this means.

Therefore, I deeply appreciate Dr. Wilson's discussion of what we can do to keep as cognitively sharp as possible. I am working to follow his advice. For both professional and personal reasons, I wholeheartedly recommend this brief but important book to you.

Dr. Neil S. Glickman, Ph.D.
Licensed Clinical Psychologist
University of Massachusetts Medical School
Adjunct Professor
Author and editor of six books on
deaf mental health care

INTRODUCTION

The summer of 2019 was one to remember. Of course, the following summer might have made 2019 that much fonder. Isn't it funny how such a negative historical event as the coronavirus shelter-in-place train wreck that wreaked havoc on all of our lives can make something fonder?

That summer of 2019, my wife, three children (aged 9, 7, and 4) and I jumped into our packed family van and set out for a week-long road trip. Our travels followed a loop, initiating on a south-by-southeast trend from our home in the Pacific Northwest through the Rocky Mountains of Utah, turning northward to trek through the beautiful vistas of Wyoming before finally returning westward home.

Among the highlights of the trip was a stop to visit a lesser-known locale called Legend Rock, an archaeology site containing beautiful ancient rock artworks. This petroglyph site is located approximately thirty miles northwest of Thermopolis, Wyoming, a quaint town legendary for its numerous mineral hot springs. Getting to Legend Rock requires traveling an off-road circuitous, desert-like, and dusty route.

Upon arrival at the visitor's center, we were greeted by a cheerful elderly woman outfitted in a full-brim hat, tan button-up polo, dark green shorts, and sturdy hiking shoes. She introduced herself as a volunteer ranger before proceeding to explain the special rules for hiking the Legend Rock trail.

Although I do not remember all of the rules cited, two rules stood out: first, to not touch any of the petroglyph panels, and second, to not to kick up dust while hiking near the vertical cliff wall containing the etched rock art. I don't know why these two rules stood out, but it may have had something to do with the fleeting panic I felt at the thought of my wife and me trying to keep our little herd in order. "Keep the dust down! Don't touch the rock! No, that's not the place to go to the bathroom!" My thoughts were confirmed at the sight of our kids already jumping over the nearby picnic tables, running circles around us, giddy with excitement to finally be out of their seatbelts and on stable ground.

The revelation of the rules from the ranger required a parental game plan. My wife and I huddled together to draw up our plan of attack. We decided the best strategy was to leverage our baby carrier backpack. I would carry our four-year-old on my back until we at least finished viewing the panels and were at a safe distance from the fragile rock art. That would free up my hands to take on another child while my wife took the other. Man-to-man coverage at its finest. We broke our huddle and proceeded to execute the plan.

As we traipsed from the visitor center toward the trailhead, my wife and I noted several signs alerting hikers to be wary of rattlesnakes. We wasted nary a second letting our two on-the-ground children know about the potential dangers lurking in the brush or under rocks. The warning didn't serve as the ammo to stay as close to us as I hoped it would—at least not for a seven-year-old boy who took to the news like a horse to grain. His curiosity piqued as his eyes immediately began scanning the fields for a slithering animal. The clear body language was all I needed to grab his hand and hang on to it until he pleaded with a promise to stay on the trail near us.

The combination of being on solid ground, breathing in fresh air, and taking in the beautiful mid-morning sunshine was a reward in itself. It was a surprisingly short hike to the vertical cliffs where the ancient artwork tantalizes the imagination in all its over-11,000-year-old glory. Although some panels had eroded over the centuries and were barely visible to the naked eye, it was fascinating to peruse these last vestiges of precious records giving us a glimpse of what life was like all those many years ago.

After snapping the requisite family photos (yes, we managed to get our little herd to pose for 0.023 of a second), we started to make our way back to the van. By this time, the sun was high in the sky, pushing the mercury mercilessly to an uncomfortable level. The miserable heat reached the point where my nine-year-old daughter asked if I could add her as a passenger on my body. I proceeded to carry both of my girls as we trekked the thankfully short hike back to our van.

As a board-certified neuropsychologist, I couldn't help but see the multiple parallels between the window into history afforded by the petroglyph panels and our personal memories. The visible quality of the various panels could be considered as part of a continuum. On one side of the continuum were clearly visible artwork pieces. On the opposite side were pieces that were nearly faded or even conspicuously chiseled out by a daring poacher.

Our personal memories could also be considered as part of a continuum. Depending on one's neurological status at any given time, individuals may have normal memory functions with no noticeable dysfunction. Deteriorations in memory functions may be noted for individuals with a given neurological injury.

Folks who know me understand that I have a great appreciation for metaphors and the insights representative symbols can bring to the abstract. The metaphor that I saw at Legend Rock was this: Much like we can take action to protect the ancient petroglyph panels, we can protect another, very personal form of history—our brains. There are certain things we can do as we age to protect our brains to allow ourselves to enjoy life to the fullest and for the longest time possible.

Instead of dust kicked up by hikers passing by or the oily residue left on the artwork by prying human fingers, the enemy that erodes our personal memories is dementia.

PART I: **DEMENTIA DEFINED AND THE FOUR MOST COMMON TYPES**

Just as there are various methods of erosion that ancient petroglyphs can undergo, such as oily residue from human touch, excess dust, or water, the human mind can be subject to multiple paths of cognitive decline. Such diverse ways have different prognoses and treatment courses. We begin our journey into the symbolic etchings of the mind by defining what comprises dementia and how this compares to normal aging. A discussion on differentiating the four most common dementia types then follows.

CHAPTER ONE
WHAT IS DEMENTIA AND IS IT A NORMAL PART OF AGING?

"We'll be friends until we're old and senile.
Then we'll be new friends."
Author Unknown

Did you know that dementia afflicts 32% of individuals aged 85 years or older?[1] Looking at this statistic a different way, this reflects approximately one-third of the world population. That's a lot of individuals. In fact, you and I have probably met or know someone with dementia.

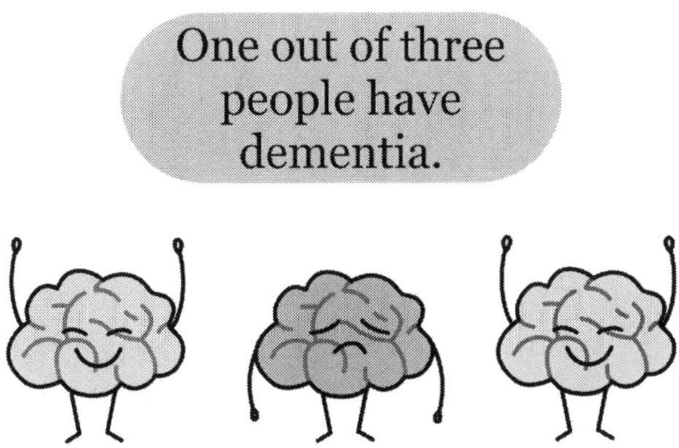

Dementia is an umbrella term that describes a set of symptoms impairing memory or the ability to think clearly. Later in this book, we will discuss different types of dementia with which an individual might present (eg, Alzheimer's disease). In addition to cognitive decline, personality changes or language dysfluency may be observed.[2,3]

As you can imagine, when memory or the ability to think clearly is impaired, there are repercussions to one's life. Individuals may no longer be able to engage in typical daily activities. Basic everyday routines are disrupted. Driving, cooking a meal, or managing the bills becomes challenging. Witnessing such functional declines can be devastating to the spouse, partner, family members, and friends.

As the quote on page 3 attests, there are doubtless occasions that could be included under one's "funny memories about life" journal. Preceding each chapter throughout this book, you will see quotes that invite laughter without any intention of poking fun at the debilitation associated with dementia. You will also read the occasional facetious story of family members, caretakers, friends, or my own personal and professional experiences working with individuals with dementia. These quotes and stories are meant to help us in maintaining equanimity and perspective as we learn together. After all, research shows that we tend to remember more if we're having fun while we learn. (And there goes our first tip for enhancing memory.)

Before we progress further, let's look back at the question that is the second part of this chapter's heading: Is dementia considered a normal part of aging?

If you answered no, you are correct. Dementia is not a normal part of aging and shouldn't be part of the expectations of the so-called golden years of life. You might be thinking to yourself, but it seems that many elderly folks I know experience some kind of cognitive decline. . . aren't these dementia symptoms? While we all experience decline in certain areas of brain function as we age, these declines do not rise to the level of impairment that entails dementia per se.

What Declines as the Brain Ages?

Now that we have busted the myth of dementia being a normal part of aging, let's tackle another question: what exactly is considered a normal part of aging?

Anatomical and imaging studies of the brain across the life span have revealed differences in brain structure, though not everyone has the exact same volume of brain changes in the exact same areas of the brain. Generally speaking, however, the greatest areas of shrinkage are found in the areas of the caudate, cerebellum, hippocampus, white matter tracts, and tertiary association cortices.[4,5] The functions of these anatomical brain areas are explained further below.

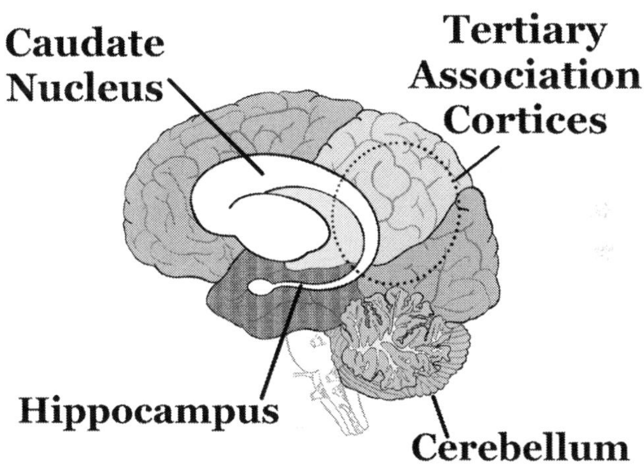

Caudate: Is involved in automatic learned behaviors.[6] For example, we may have driven a manual stick transmission since our teenage years and internalized the timing of shifting the gears. As the caudate declines, the likelihood of our automatic learned behaviors taking over declines, increasing the risks of mistakes such as leaving an engine over-revving or even lugging in the wrong gear for too long.

Cerebellum: Coordinates voluntary movements such as posture, balance, signing, and speech. The cerebellum helps with smooth muscular movement. There is also evidence that the cerebellum may play at least a minor role in cognition, behavior, and psychiatric illness.[7]

Hippocampus: Is involved in learning as well as the formation of new memories. The hippocampus also plays a significant role in the consolidation of new memories.[8] Consolidation is the process of transferring the memory to long-term storage.

Tertiary Association Cortices: Integrates and coordinates visual, auditory, and sensory information.[9] Vision, hearing, touch, taste, and smell are within this purview.

White Matter Tracts: More on this below.

You may wonder, "So, what does all of the shrinkage in these areas of the brain mean?" It all comes down to this: as we age, we may struggle more with free recall of information (especially newly acquired information), but recognition retrieval remains intact.[10-12] That means that older individuals may not do as well as their younger counterparts on short-answer exams where free recall is in heavy demand. However, when cues are provided—such as on multiple choice exams—our intact recognition retrieval functions kick in and our performance rises to the level of young adults.

Does Youth Reign Omnipotent in Terms of Memory Advantages?

Fortunately, no. Not all is doom and gloom for older individuals in terms of memory functions. In fact, we rival, and even exceed, our young adult counterparts in some areas of memory performance. For example, once we have put in the requisite time studying and digesting information we've aimed to learn, we are less likely to forget the learned information.[13-15] Now that's an area that us older individuals can boast about. (*So there! Take that, young punks!*)

Oh, and let's not forget about the white matter tracts referenced earlier. White matter tracts are the axons and wires in the brain

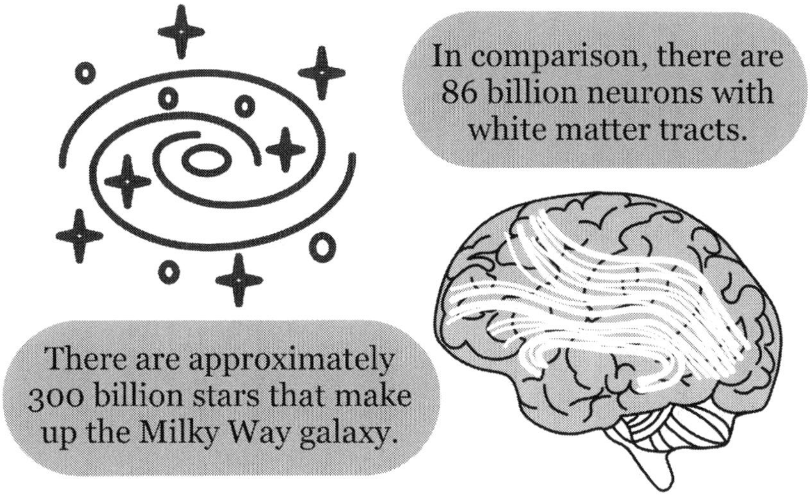

that transmit information to different structures in the cerebral cortex. These white matter tracts tend to decrease with advancing age.[16] The decrease in white matter is the reason older adults may show selective losses in functions related to speed and efficiency of information processing.

I am always floored when I consider the comparison of the brain's neurons to the stars of our Milky Way galaxy. The brain has roughly one-third the number of neurons as stars in our home galaxy. There are roughly 300 billion stars in the Milky Way galaxy compared to about 86 billion neurons in the brain. Recall that white matter fibers (axons) are extensions of these neurons. These are a lot of white matter tracts.

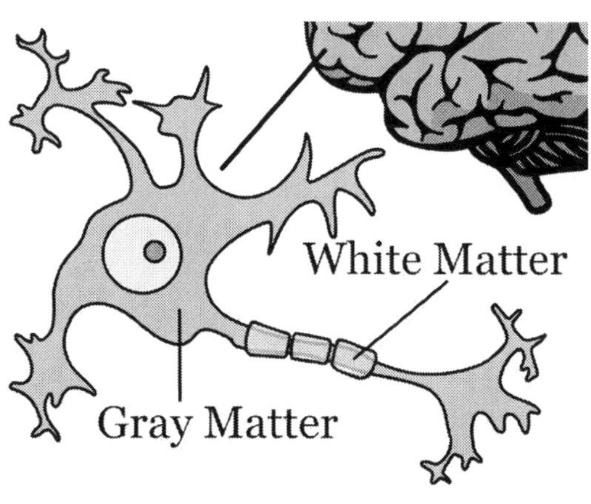

Decreased white matter is thought to be brought on by perfusion disturbances in blood vessels throughout the brain.[17,18] As the supply of oxygen in blood vessels decreases, white matter tends to die off or vanish. If there is a severe blockage in the flow of blood to the brain, it can lead to infarction, or death of gray matter.

But what exactly is cortical gray matter? Gray matter is the thinking part of the brain. You can think of it as the computer (or central processing unit [CPU]) part of the brain. These gray matter parts are essentially the brain's nerve cells.

Most dementias arise from problems associated with the nerve cells of the brain associated with memory functioning. The gray matter essentially becomes nonfunctional and shrinks, leading to reductions in overall gray matter. However, in normal aging, gray matter for important areas of memory functioning remains relatively unchanged, as shown in the illustration on the previous page.[19]

Interestingly, one popular myth is that the size of the brain is correlated with a higher IQ. (If this myth were true, males would tend to be smarter than females, which we know is not true!) It is not a larger brain that is associated with a higher IQ. Rather, it is the density of gray matter that is correlated with IQ.[20]

What Age Is Older and Is It Dementia or Ordinary Forgetfulness?

A common question is, "At what age am I considered 'older'?" Most of the significant changes to the brain described above tend to occur when people are in their 60s. It is generally after the age of 65 that we might consider ourselves as being within the third age or the golden years.

Another question that people sometimes ask is about what Alzheimer's or other dementia conditions can look like and how this is different from ordinary forgetfulness (otherwise known as the almost daily "Where did I put my keys?" occurrence). Memory difficulties most critically involve recent events.[21] While some forgetfulness is a normal characteristic of being human, it is important to understand that with Alzheimer's, especially in the early stages, things that an individual normally could do independently start becoming problematic.

For instance, an individual with early-stage Alzheimer's may start requiring help with once-routine activities such as paying bills, grocery shopping, or driving to various places. When someone begins to need help with daily living, such as dressing, bathing, or other basic life functions, this should raise concern. It is usually at this stage that help should be sought from an appropriate healthcare provider.

It is also just as important to recognize that not everyone with mild cognitive impairment has Alzheimer's. There are a variety of healthcare conditions that can contribute to states of mild cognitive impairment that have absolutely no correlation with a true dementia condition. Examples of health conditions that can mimic dementia include dehydration, hypothyroidism, bacteriuria (also known as a urinary tract infection or UTI), nutritional deficiencies (lack of vitamin B12), or vector-borne infections (such as West Nile Virus, Lyme Disease, malaria). Close to 40% of individuals who show signs of a dementia condition may actually be suffering from an undetected illness that is treatable and modifiable.[22] This is part of the reason it is important to follow up with a healthcare provider.

Key Takeaways

I am delighted that you have chosen to join me in this incredible journey through the inner workings of our amazing brain. As you read at the beginning of this chapter, *the etchings of the mind* is a metaphor meant to convey that just as there are steps that can be taken to protect ancient petroglyph panels, there are certain things that we can do to protect the personal historical record that exists in our brains.

If ancient rock carvings are appropriately protected, they can be preserved over the years for the visual enjoyment of many. The same ideas of longevity apply to the human brain. Under normal conditions, the brain should remain vital and healthy for a lifetime. The myth that dementia is a normal part of aging is just that—a myth.

While normal aging does present some decrements in certain neuroanatomical areas of the brain, we older individuals still have some advantages over our younger counterparts. The biggest advantage lies in the fact that once we put in the extra time to learn information, we are less likely to forget the information.

As we get into the golden years (over the age of 65), we may naturally start to wonder or even worry about lapses in memory functions we might experience as we go about our daily lives. The following table summarizes the differences you might see between normal aging and a potential dementia condition. That said, it is always important to follow up with a healthcare provider to rule out dementia as well as other conditions that can mimic dementia.

Normal Aging	Potential Dementia Condition
Forgetting to pay a bill one month	Difficulties with routine tasks on an ongoing basis (eg, bills, driving, taking medications)
Drawing a blank on a person's name	When loved ones notice memory loss before you do
Occasionally misplacing personal items	Neglecting to take care of oneself, such as not bathing or eating poorly
Making more lists to remember tasks	Repeating the same question or conversation, over and over
Sporadic "tip-of-the-tongue" phenomenon	Frequent pauses to retrieve words and memories
Looking for your car in the parking lot	Getting lost in familiar places or withdrawing from social activities

CHAPTER ONE REFERENCES

1. Alzheimer's disease facts and figures. *Alzheimers Dement.* 2020;16(3):391-460.
2. Haak NJ. Maintaining connections: Understanding communication from the perspective of persons with dementia. *Alzheimers Care Today.* 2002;3(2):116-131.
3. Blair M, Marczinski CA, Davis-Faroque N, Kertesz A. A longitudinal study of language decline in Alzheimer's disease and frontotemporal dementia. *J Int Neuropsychol Soc.* 2007;13(2):237-245.
4. Raz N, Lindenberger U, Rodrigue KM, et al. Regional brain changes in aging healthy adults: general trends, individual differences and modifiers. *Cereb Cortex.* 2005;15(11):1676-1689.
5. Raz N, Ghisletta P, Rodrigue KM, Kennedy KM, Lindenberger U. Trajectories of brain aging in middle-aged and older adults: regional and individual differences. *Neuroimage.* 2010;51(2):501-511.
6. Chiu Y-C, Jiang J, Egner T. The caudate nucleus mediates learning of stimulus–control state associations. *J Neurosci.* 2017;37(4):1028-1038.
7. Rapoport M, van Reekum R, Mayberg H. The role of the cerebellum in cognition and behavior: a selective review. *J Neuropsychiatry Clin Neurosci.* 2000;12(2):193-198.
8. Wittenberg GM, Tsien JZ. An emerging molecular and cellular framework for memory processing by the hippocampus. *Trends Neurosci.* 2002;25(10):501-505.
9. Harrison DW. Functional cortical levels within units 2 and 3. *Brain Asymmetry and Neural Systems.* Springer; 2015:45-52.
10. Davis HP, Small SA, Stern Y, Mayeux R, Feldstein SN, Keller FR. Acquisition, recall, and forgetting of verbal information in long-term memory by young, middle-aged, and elderly individuals. *Cortex.* 2003;39(4-5):1063-1091.
11. Balota DA, Dolan PO, Duchek JM. Memory changes in healthy young and older adults. *The Oxford Handbook of Memory.* 2000:395-410.

12. Luo L, Craik FI. Aging and memory: a cognitive approach. *Can J Psychiatry.* 2008;53(6):346-353. doi:10.1177/070674370805300603
13. Willis SL, Jones R, Ball, K, et al. *Advanced Cognitive Training for Independent and Vital Elderly (ACTIVE), United States, 1999-2008.* Inter-university Consortium for Political and Social Research; 2015. doi:10.3886/ICPSR36036.v1
14. Zhao Y, Tudorascu DL, Lopez OL, et al. Amyloid β deposition and suspected non-Alzheimer pathophysiology and cognitive decline patterns for 12 years in oldest old participants without dementia. *JAMA Neurol.* 2018;75(1):88-96.
15. Verssimo J, Verhaeghen P, Goldman N, Weinstein M, Ullman MT. Evidence that aging yields improvements as well as declines across attention and executive functions. *Nat Hum Behav.* 2021:1-14.
16. Coelho A, Fernandes HM, Magalhães R, et al. Signatures of white-matter microstructure degradation during aging and its association with cognitive status. *Sci Rep.* 2021;11(1):1-12.
17. ten Dam VH, van den Heuvel DM, de Craen AJ, et al. Decline in total cerebral blood flow is linked with increase in periventricular but not deep white matter hyperintensities. *Radiology.* 2007;243(1):198-203.
18. Gunning-Dixon FM, Raz N. The cognitive correlates of white matter abnormalities in normal aging: a quantitative review. *Neuropsychology.* 2000;14(2):224.
19. Hafkemeijer A, Altmann-Schneider I, de Craen AJ, Slagboom PE, van der Grond J, Rombouts SA. Associations between age and gray matter volume in anatomical brain networks in middle-aged to older adults. *Aging Cell.* 2014;13(6):1068-1074.
20. Narr KL, Woods RP, Thompson PM, et al. Relationships between IQ and regional cortical gray matter thickness in healthy adults. *Cereb Cortex.* 2007;17(9):2163-2171.
21. Leyhe T, Müller S, Milian M, Eschweiler GW, Saur R. Impairment of episodic and semantic autobiographical memory in patients with mild cognitive impairment and early Alzheimer's disease. *Neuropsychologia.* 2009;47(12):2464-2469.

22. Hodgson N, Gitlin LN, Winter L, Czekanski K. Undiagnosed illness and neuropsychiatric behaviors in community-residing older adults with dementia. *Alzheimer Dis Assoc Disord.* 2011;25(2):109.

CHAPTER TWO
THE FOUR MOST COMMON TYPES OF DEMENTIA

In the first chapter, we discussed the prevalence of dementia (nearly one-third of the world population). The widespread prevalence of dementia definitely isn't helped by the fact that there are over 100 different types of dementia or conditions that can impede memory or the ability to think clearly. In this chapter, we will focus on the four most common dementias from most to least prevalent:

1. Alzheimer's disease
2. Vascular dementia
3. Lewy body dementia
4. Frontotemporal dementia.

The Most Common Dementia: Alzheimer's Disease

Alzheimer's disease occurs in approximately 50-75% of all dementia cases.[1-3] Also, the majority of cases of Alzheimer's develop after age 65.[4,5] The number of cases significantly increases across the seventh (2%), eighth (6%), and ninth (50+%) decades of life.

An Alzheimer's disease diagnosis after age 65 is classified as "late onset." Late onset Alzheimer's tends to have a slow and insidious course, lasting approximately 10+ years.[8]

The minority of Alzheimer's cases that occur before the age of 65 are referenced as "early onset." Early onset Alzheimer's often demonstrates a stronger genetic etiology.[9,10] Early onset has a more rapid progression.

Behavior Symptoms of Alzheimer's

Patients in the early stages of Alzheimer's will often minimize cognitive problems and may confabulate information, which could lead to easily overlooking actual memory deficits.[11] For example, if you happen to ask someone what he or she had for breakfast, a plausible response could be bacon and eggs or cereal. Unless you are living with the individual and actually saw what they ate for breakfast, you would not know that the response was incorrect.

As the disease progresses, other symptoms become more apparent, such as agitation, confusion, wandering, apathy, decreased sleep and appetite, and emotional blunting. Delusions and hallucinations can also occur in the late stages of Alzheimer's.

Pathophysiology of Alzheimer's

To understand the pathophysiology of Alzheimer's within the brain, we have to look at the cellular level. After all, it is the decay and death of the cells of the brain that result in the overall shrinkage of the cerebral cortex that is often seen on autopsy of an individual with Alzheimer's. Cellular injury and its subsequent death begin with the compilation of a plaque-forming protein called *beta-amyloid*.

Beta-amyloid forms when secretase enzymes cut off the tail and head from proteins on the external cell surface. You can think of secretase as being similar to scissors, while enzymes are catalysts that bring about biochemical reactions in the body. The alpha-secretase enzyme cuts the short form of the protein 90-95% of the time. The long form of the protein is cut by the beta-secretase enzyme. While normal brains may have 5-10% beta-amyloid, in Alzheimer's brains it is at 40%.[12,13]

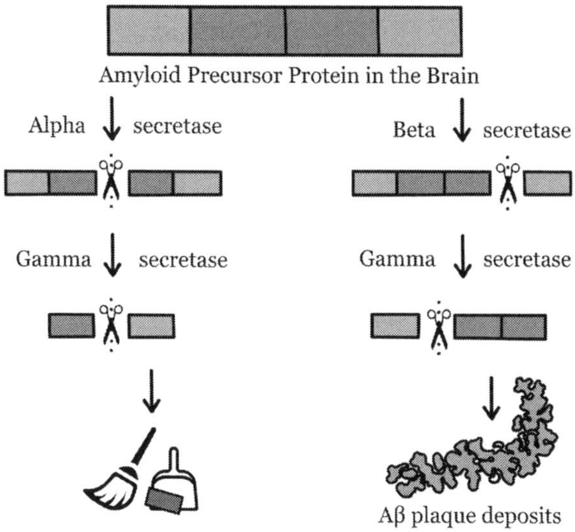

Beta-amyloid tends to be marked for destruction by small "tags" referred to as *ubiquitin.* The brain, unfortunately, cannot carry out the metabolic destruction of excess levels of beta-amyloid. Only small amounts (5-10%) of beta-amyloid can be cleared from the brain.

The excess beta-amyloid that cannot be carried out by the brain forms a dense core on the surface of the neuron or cell. These excess beta-amyloid proteins activate *microglia* (a macrophage that removes damaged neurons) and *reactive astrocytes* (regulates immune responses). The activation invites a *phagocytic* (cell destroying) clearance of the excess beta-amyloid, which in turn, obliterates otherwise healthy cells.

The destructive nature of the phagocytic clearance of the beta-amyloid proteins leaves behind degenerated cells, dendrites, and axons. The broken-down connections between networks of neurons results in widespread loss of brain volume. This is the reason patients with Alzheimer's often evidence a shrunken or atrophied brain on autopsy.[14]

The destruction of healthy cells is also known as *apoptosis.* Cell apoptosis is essentially the process that leads to neuronal cell death. The concept of cell apoptosis is believed to account for the pathophysiology of several neurodegenerative diseases outside of Alzheimer's, including amyotrophic lateral sclerosis (Lou Gehrig's disease), spinal muscular atrophy, and Parkinson's disease.

As the beta-amyloid plaque multiplies over time, symptoms become worse, and it becomes harder for people to remember recent events, reason, or recognize people they know. Tau protein—which serves as the cell's internal skeleton—also becomes hyperphosphorylated, resulting in a twisted filament referenced in the scientific literature as neurofibrillary tangles.

The easiest way to envision neurofibrillary tangles is to consider what happens when you have multiple electronic items plugged into a single power strip. Often these electronic wires become entangled into a big eyesore chunk that can be a hassle to untangle. It is essentially the same thing that occurs in the brain—the neurons and axons (or electronic wires) start to degenerate, losing the ability to maintain their original shape. The loss of the original shape results in the neurofibrillary tangles.

In addition to multiplying beta-amyloid plaques, one of the main brain chemicals—referenced in scientific parlance as a

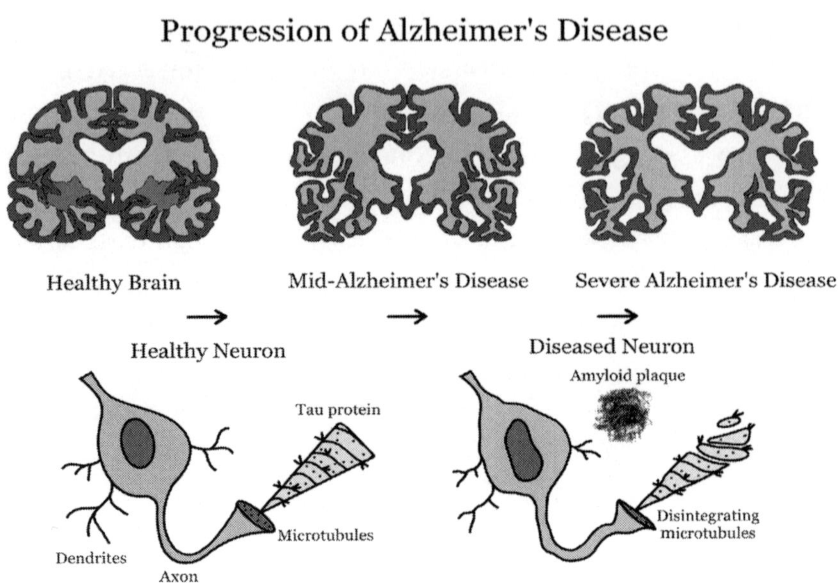

neurotransmitter—that is depleted in Alzheimer's is acetylcholine. Acetylcholine is responsible for maintaining short-term memory, attention, executive functioning, and novelty seeking.

The brain area where acetylcholine is produced has an interesting name: *nucleus basalis of Meynert*. The nucleus basalis of Meynert is located in the basal forebrain area and is the structure containing a high density of acetylcholine neurons. When acetylcholine is depleted, the symptoms of Alzheimer's are apparent with compromise of memory and executive functioning.

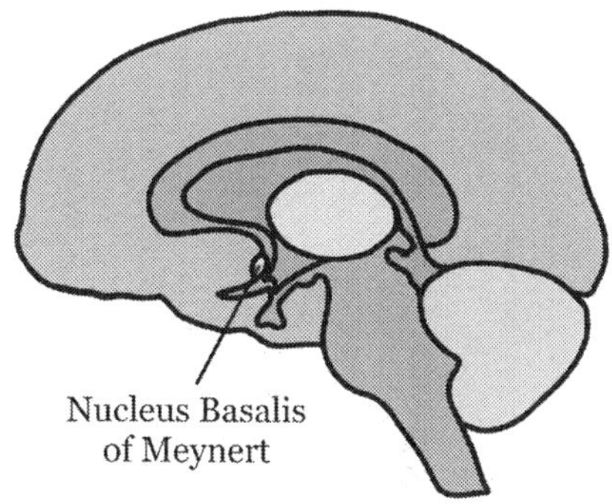

There are genetic conditions that may increase the risk of an individual developing Alzheimer's. For example, apolipoprotein E (apoE) is a glycoprotein that transports cholesterol in the blood. The apoE glycoprotein also plays a role in cellular repair. An allele of the apoE gene, known as E4, increases the risk of Alzheimer's and is associated with deficits on chromosome 19.[15] ApoE-E4 interferes with the removal of beta-amyloid from the extracellular space.

Beta-amyloid is believed to be associated with mutations on chromosome 21. The story behind the identification of the beta-amyloid chromosome's association to Alzheimer's disease is fascinating. Given that the brains of individuals with Down syndrome, which is caused by an extra 21st chromosome (or trisomy 21), also contain deposits of beta-amyloid, neuroscientists began to wonder if the 21st chromosome may have an association with Alzheimer's. It turns out that chromosome 21 does, in fact, contain the gene that produces the Alzheimer's disease generating beta-amyloid.[16] The finding of beta-amyloid associated with chromosome 21 is part of the reason Alzheimer's is frequently seen in individuals with Down syndrome.

Paradoxically, for all of the evils of beta-amyloid, research also indicates that the physiological role of beta-amyloid protein may include functions that allow it to act as a sealant at sites of injury or leakage of brain blood vessel walls.[17,18] Yes, you read that right — beta-amyloid protein isn't all as malicious as we've made it sound.

Evidence further indicates that beta-amyloid may have antimicrobial (kills foreign or bad bacteria) functions.[19] Although there remains much research to confirm the functions of beta-amyloid, it appears that they do have positive functions of both blood vessel repair and antimicrobial actions. As with most things in life, too much of anything can be bad. This golden rule of life applies in terms of the excess accumulation of beta-amyloid protein leading to the onset of Alzheimer's.

Before we move on to the second most common dementia, it is important to understand that dementia conditions, not just Alzheimer's, are frequently involved with an inflammatory response in the brain.[17] In the case of Alzheimer's, the beta-amyloid aggregates activate an inflammatory response that triggers the release of chemicals produced by the immune system that normally destroy infected cells. These chemicals, referenced as toxic cytokines, trigger excess release of a neurotransmitter called glutamate. Excess release of glutamate creates too much stimulation (excitotoxicity) of nerve receptors in the brain, damaging them in the process. The resulting damage leads to further cognitive, emotional, and physical declines in day-to-day functioning.

The Second Most Common Dementia: Vascular Dementia

Vascular dementia occurs in 20-30% of cases. As individuals age, the risk for vascular problems (eg, strokes) increases. This increase in the potential for vascular problems parallels the increase in risk for development of vascular dementia.[18]

Onset of vascular dementia typically occurs between 60 to 75 years of age.[19] The course of vascular dementia varies based on the different sizes and locations of ischemic events within the brain.[20] An ischemic event happens when there is an inadequate blood supply to the brain or any organ of the body, such as the heart.

Many vascular dementia cases progress in a stepwise manner, with periods of stability followed by rapid deterioration due to additional strokes. The stepwise course can sometimes be difficult to identify and may appear to present as "continuously progressive."[21]

Other cases can progress slowly and gradually. These slower and more gradual cases may not be noticed by patients or their loved ones. Neuropsychological or neuroimaging studies may pick up on such subtleties. For example, with neuropsychological exams, differences in pure motor functions between the left and right side of the body may be noted. Neuropsychological exams can also reveal a data profile that maps onto individuals with a vascular dementia presentation. With neuroimaging studies, multiple remote ("old") ischemic events may be identified or noted.

Behavior Symptoms of Vascular Dementia

The clinical presentation of vascular dementia can vary widely, depending on the site of the stroke and penumbra (shadow of affected area) within the brain. Neurological signs and symptoms can range from minimal to severe. Consider, for example, a stroke that occurs in a specific area of the primary motor cortex. There may be fine motor coordination issues, gait and balance problems, unilateral (one-sided) motor deficits, sensory deficits, spasticity, or rigidity. Symptoms of depression and anxiety are also common. Urinary incontinence may be present.

Another example of the wide variation in clinical presentation that can be seen might be an ischemic lesion to the bilateral parietal-occipital lobes or even only the parietal or occipital lobe alone. Ischemic lesions in these areas can result in a phenomenon known as Bálint's syndrome.[22]

Given the association of the parietal-occipital areas with the spatial and visual centers of the brain, it makes sense that observed symptoms in Bálint's syndrome can include a visuoconstructional apraxia. An example of a visuoconstructional apraxia would be the inability to copy a simple geometric design.

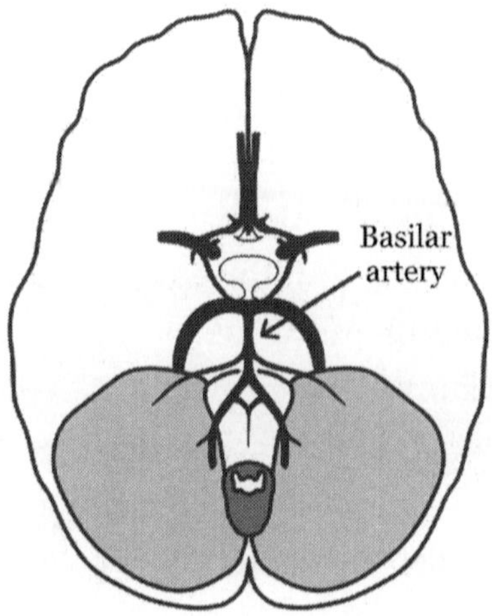

Bálint's syndrome is also associated with various visual problems related to the inability to move the eyes as desired. For example, ocular apraxia (the inability to scan extrapersonal space with the eyes) or optic ataxia (dysmetric or saccadic jerks that can result in blurred vision) may occur. A phenomenon referred to as simultanagnosia may also be noted, which is an inability to perceive a scene with multiple parts to it. Although the patient with simultanagnosia has a normal visual field, they can only see and recognize an individual element of a scene, being unable to perceive the overall picture.

Not only does Bálint's syndrome manifest with visual-spatial problems, it can also be accompanied by another syndrome known as Gerstmann's syndrome.[23,24] Gerstmann's syndrome is characterized by the loss of four specific neurological functions: 1) Inability to write (dysgraphia or agraphia); 2) Loss of the ability to do calculations (acalculia); 3) Difficulties or inability identifying one's own or another's fingers (finger agnosia); and 4) Inability to make the distinction between the right and left side of the body. It is rare for a person to experience all four neurological dysfunctions at once. In the Bálint's syndrome manifestation of

Gerstmann's, the dominant parietal lobe is affected in the area of the angular gyrus.

Ischemic lesions to the parietal-occipital lobes or either lobe alone may be due to *basilar artery occlusion,* the closing off of the artery. An illustration of the anatomy of the basilar artery is on the previous page, which shows the brain underside's midsection.

A basilar artery occlusion—sometimes referred to as "top of the basilar syndrome"—can also result in infarction (tissue injury or death) of the thalamus, midbrain, and parts of the temporal lobes.[25] Noted behavioral symptoms include delirium, peduncular hallucinosis (brain stem-induced visual hallucinations), obtundation (diminished alertness), and memory deficits. Problems with controlling eye movement (visual gaze palsy) or involuntary repetitive eye movements (nystagmus) may also occur.

Pathophysiology of Vascular Dementia

Vascular dementia is caused by small strokes in the brain.[26] A stroke occurs when the flow of oxygen through blood vessels is decreased or even blocked. The lack of sufficient blood flow results in an infarction which, as noted above, is irreversible death of localized tissue at the site of the stroke. When the cumulative effects of tissue damage to various areas within the brain, such as white matter tracts or neurons, reach a certain level, symptoms of vascular dementia may surface.

There are several different types of strokes. The most common types of strokes can be described as occurring from hemorrhagic, ischemic, or atherosclerotic events.[27] In a hemorrhagic stroke, a weakened blood vessel wall ruptures, resulting in bleeding within the brain. Due to the hemorrhage, necessary blood and oxygen to vital areas of the brain are drastically reduced.

An ischemic stroke occurs when there is an obstruction within a blood vessel. It can occur from a blood clot which results in thrombus (partial blockage) or emboli (full blockage) of the blood vessel. The obstruction results in decreased perfusion or hypoxia, which is a deficiency of oxygen to meet the needs of the brain tissue. Depending on where in the brain the blockage occurs, behavioral manifestations and symptoms will vary.

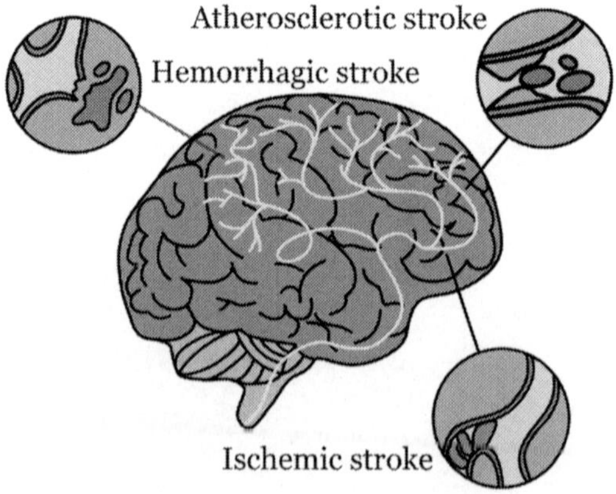

The final most common stroke event occurs as a result of atherosclerosis, which occurs due to plaque or build up in an artery. The buildup within the artery creates an obstruction that reduces blood flow to areas of the brain. The reduced blood flow can result in death to the myelinated axons of neurons (known as white matter tract infarcts). Recall that myelinated axons are the white matter tracts that speed up the relaying of information to different parts of the brain.

Early identification of vascular dementia symptoms is crucial for effective treatment. Neuroimaging does not always identify vascular dementia symptoms. Sometimes ischemic strokes may be too small for visible identification on traditional neuroimaging.[28] In these cases, neuropsychological examinations can be beneficial for early diagnosis. Without clinical findings from a comprehensive neuropsychological exam, neuroimaging can be misleading, resulting in a false negative (results that appear to be normal when it should not be).[29,30]

Another symptom of vascular dementia that can present is what is called Babinski's sign (also known as an extensor plantar response).[34] Babinski's sign occurs when the sole of the foot is firmly stroked and the big toe moves upward while the other toes fan out. This sign or reflex is normal in children up to age two.

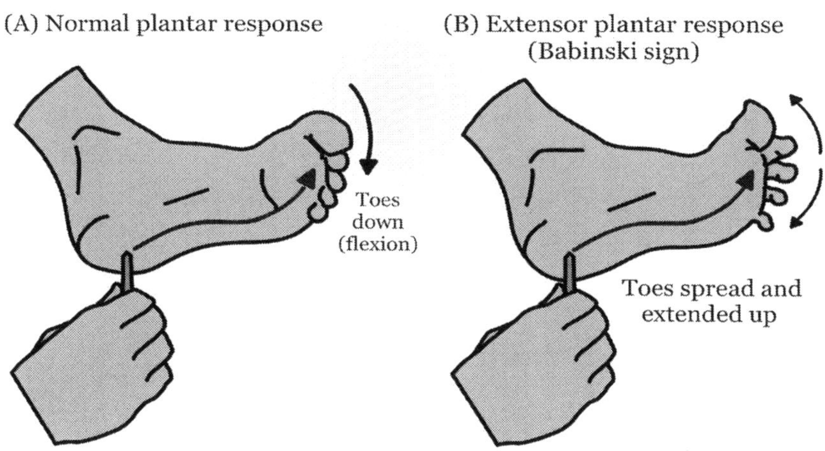

When Babinski's reflex occurs in a child older than age two or in an adult, it is often a sign of vascular dementia.

However, Babinski's reflex can also be a sign of another type of central nervous system disorder that involves a lesion somewhere within the brain and spinal cord. Examples of other disorders that can have a positive Babinski's sign include amyotrophic lateral sclerosis (aka Lou Gehrig's disease), brain tumor, meningitis (an infection of the membranes covering the spinal cord), multiple sclerosis, or a stroke.

Third Most Common Dementia: Dementia with Lewy Bodies

Lewy body disease or dementia is found in 10% to 25% of all cases of dementia.[31] Lewy body dementia tends to have an earlier onset than either Alzheimer's or vascular dementia. The age of onset for dementia with Lewy bodies is typically between 50 and 70 years of age.[32] The clinical presentation is punctuated by periods (hours to days) of marked fluctuation in mental status and orientation. Family members often remark on the variability in behavioral presentation and cognitive fluctuation when describing observed behavioral deficits.[33] For example, the affected individual may not recognize a familiar face one day, but then return to normal recognition the next day.

Patients who experience a rapid decline with sudden changes in cognition can leave loved ones and caregivers grasping for ways to adjust and find help. Steep and quick declines in functioning can be extremely stressful for individuals closest to the patient with Lewy body dementia.

Behavior Symptoms of Lewy Body Dementia

One of the prominent features of Lewy body dementia is visual hallucinations. Such hallucinations can be frightening to the individual experiencing them. Sometimes visual hallucinations can be initiated through misinterpretation of an actual object in the visual field.

There is real-life video footage accessible via YouTube of an elderly male with dementia with Lewy bodies.[34] The individual can be seen actively experiencing hallucinations that involve misinterpretation of objects (in this case, the dust on the floor misinterpreted as "big black bugs with red flowers on them") as well as visual hallucinations.

Visual hallucinations brought on by dementia with Lewy bodies can be frightening for both the patient and their caretakers. Hallucinations can be clear and well-formed, creating the perception of a realistic sensory experience.[35] These realistic hallucinatory symptoms can elicit behaviors that may endanger the patient or caretaker(s).

As an example of how the hallucinations can engender potentially problematic behaviors, the aforementioned video of the individual who saw the clear and well-formed "big black bugs" perceived these creatures as trying to steal personal effects, including the refrigerator. At one point, in attempting to prevent the refrigerator from being stolen, the individual almost pulled the refrigerator on top of himself.

An interesting phenomenon is when the hallucination symptoms involve visions of people. The visual hallucinations of people mostly appear small in size (or similar to children). The aforementioned video footage link contains this type of hallucinatory experience towards the end of the clip.

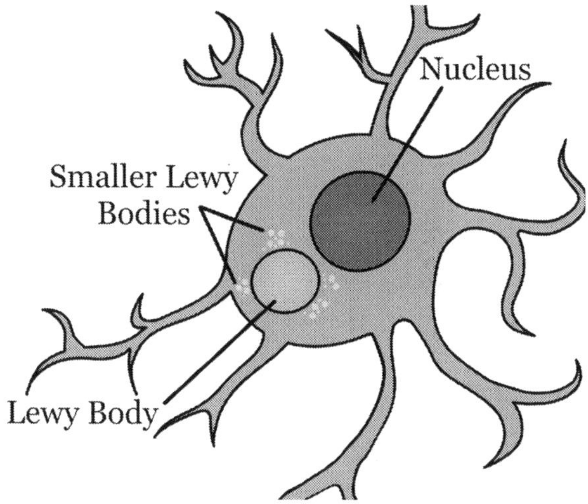

Flailing or violent movements during sleep are another possible behavioral symptom of dementia with Lewy bodies. These movements during sleep are known in the scientific literature as Rapid Eye Movement (REM) behavior sleep disorder, which involves an absence of normal REM sleep paralysis. Individuals with REM sleep behavior disorder act out their dreams by hitting, kicking, thrashing, or screaming.[36,37] They can potentially harm anyone else in bed with them. Dreams are often remembered after awakening.

REM sleep behavior disorder is associated with dementia with Lewy bodies in 50-80% of cases. It is important to note that REM sleep behavior disorder is also seen in other neurodegenerative disorders, such as Parkinson's disease.[38] In addition to potential REM sleep behavior disorder symptoms, loved ones may note an increased propensity towards trips or falls. These falls are not just simple falls but may be what are described as "violent" falls.

Pathophysiology of Dementia with Lewy Bodies

In scientific parlance, dementia with Lewy bodies is frequently referred to as part of a group of neurodegenerative conditions referred to as alpha-synucleinopathies (written as α-synucleinopathies). The α-synucleinopathies involve the α-synuclein protein in degenerating brain neurons.[39] Instead of a normal neuron or brain cell, small holes—termed Lewy bodies—develop on the brain cell.

Other conditions associated with the α-synucleinopathies include Parkinson's disease, multiple system atrophy, and the aforementioned REM sleep behavior disorder. Although these other disorders are associated with the group of α-synucleinopathies, dementia with Lewy bodies has a more widespread (ie, diffuse) distribution of Lewy bodies that makes it the differentiating factor from the other disorders.

A classic Lewy body is essentially a white blood cell (eosinophilic) that consists of a dense core surrounded by a halo of radiating fibers (fibrils). The primary structural component of these fibrils is α-synuclein. It is the fibrils composed of α-synuclein that are thought to mediate disruption of cellular homeostasis through its mechanism of creating small holes in the brain cells.[44]

While Lewy bodies have been noted in Alzheimer's disease and Down syndrome, both of these conditions also have the previously described beta-amyloid and tau protein deposits. The triple combination of α-synuclein, beta-amyloid, and tau protein deposits put Alzheimer's and Down syndrome in a category sometimes referred to as conditions with "triple amyloidosis."[40]

Brain cell neurodegeneration in dementia with Lewy bodies tends to occur in the right-side temporal-parietal association cortices.[41,42] This area of neurodegeneration within the right-side temporal-parietal association cortices may partly explain the visual hallucination symptoms that are a prominent feature of dementia with Lewy bodies.

Onset of dementia with Lewy bodies may be seen within 12 months of Parkinsonian motor deficits. Parkinsonian motor symptoms may be most apparent in tremors of the arms, hands, legs, or feet, with tremors decreasing or disappearing with movement. Other cardinal symptoms of Parkinsonism include bradykinesia, rigidity, balance, and gait issues.[43] Gait issues may resemble what is referenced as a "magnetic" appearance, with a marked inability to lift the feet off the floor while walking. These abnormalities may result in decreased mobility with an increased risk for falls.

In clinical settings, it can sometimes be difficult to differentiate Lewy body dementia from Parkinson's disease. Research has suggested a 12-month rule to differentiate Lewy body dementia from Parkinson's disease. If there are symptoms of Parkinson's disease noted for 12 months or longer before any cognitive impairment is noticed, then the disorder is thought to lean toward Parkinson's disease. If the time period is less than 12 months, then the disorder leans toward Lewy body dementia. In essence, Lewy body dementia tends to precede the motor signs and include visual hallucinations as well as diminished responsiveness.[44]

The how and why behind the hallucinatory symptoms in Lewy body dementia is not well understood.[44,45] Theoretically, the various holes left by Lewy bodies in the brain create gaps in communication between various neurons. The void in information from the lack of communication may cause other areas of the brain to try to fill in these gaps with other information that is not tangibly present, thus giving rise to hallucinatory symptoms.

Consider an example if you will. Imagine a farmer with Lewy body dementia looking at his horse and not being able to completely see the horse's head due to the communication gaps left by Lewy bodies between brain neurons. The farmer's brain might fill in the missing visual stimuli, with some additional, perhaps embellished, features. If the embellished feature happened to be a single pointed spiraling horn projecting from the horse's forehead (a unicorn's horn), the farmer would have quite the story to share. Could such hallucinatory symptoms have been the origin of these legendary mythical creatures?

The Fourth Most Common Dementia: Frontotemporal Dementia

The fourth most common dementia subtype occurs in 10-15% of all dementia cases. Developing earlier than the prior discussed dementias, onset of frontotemporal dementia is typically between 50 and 60 years of age. The average age of onset is 59. Development of frontotemporal dementia after age 75 is rare.[46] There are known cases of frontotemporal dementia beginning as early as 20 years of age.[47]

Gradually developing symptoms is the most common course in this type of dementia. However, once diagnosed, progression of frontotemporal dementia can be more rapid than Alzheimer's.[48] Progression generally evolves over 5 to 7 years.

Behavior Symptoms of Frontotemporal Dementia

Frontotemporal dementia has several different subtypes with the two main types being the behavioral variant and the primary progressive aphasia variant.[49-51]

In the behavioral variant of frontotemporal dementia, there are noteworthy changes to personality. Family members of individuals with frontotemporal dementia often remark that they no longer recognize their loved one for the person they once knew. It may seem as if a stranger has replaced their loved one. A flattened affect along with a seeming inability to empathize with others eventually permeates the individual's presentation. Difficulties with independently maintaining personal hygiene along with perseveration on specific topics as well as a general apathy may also be noted.

In the other frontotemporal dementia subtype, primary progressive aphasia, disruption in ease of language use creates problems for communication. These language difficulties may be noticed when speaking, signing, reading, writing, or understanding what others are saying.

Another subtype of frontotemporal dementia is Pick's disease. In addition to the usual features of frontotemporal dementia, Pick's disease can include symptoms of Kluver-Bucy syndrome. Symptoms of Kluver-Bucy include hyper-orality (excessive eating) and sensory stimulus seeking that has a compulsive quality. Inappropriate sexual behaviors can also present as part of the repertoire of troublesome behaviors.

Pathophysiology of Frontotemporal Dementia

As its name suggests, the most significant deficits with frontotemporal dementia tend to occur in the frontal lobes. The frontal lobes of the human cerebrum are responsible for a host of everyday behaviors, including but not limited to one's personality presentation. Decreased activation of the frontal lobes can result in the behavior disturbances and affect flattening described in the preceding section.

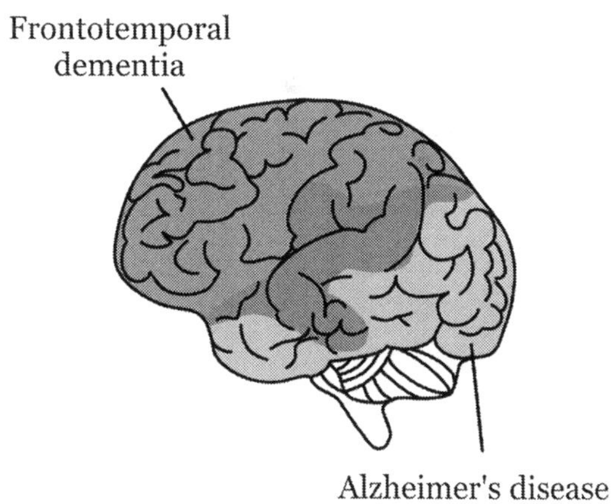

Study after study has shown that the frontal lobes determine how the brain acts on information. In essence, the relatively large size of the frontal lobes is what distinguishes our brains from other primates. A traumatic brain injury (TBI) to the frontal lobe can result in what has been described as a frontal lobe syndrome. A frontal lobe syndrome consists of slowed thinking, poor judgment, decreased curiosity, social withdrawal, and irritability.

In frontotemporal dementia, there is a build-up of defective tau proteins.[52] Recall that tau proteins normally serve as part of a cell's internal skeleton. When there is a buildup of excess tau proteins, the cell's internal skeleton is no longer properly stabilized.

The accumulation of excess tau proteins results in the spherical aggregations that appear as tiny holes burrowing into the brain tissue. Diffuse holes are localized to the frontal-temporal areas of the brain.

Key Takeaways

Whew! We have just completed an intensive journey around the four most common dementia conditions (out of over 100 different types). Given the diversity of the dementias, we have only scratched the surface with the four most common dementia types. Examples of other conditions associated with dementia include Huntington's disease, progressive supranuclear palsy (PSP), multi-system atrophy (MSA), hydrocephalus, and Creutzfeldt-Jakob disease.

For your convenience, key takeaways about the four most common dementia types are summarized below. A few reminders:

- The majority of Alzheimer's cases develop after age 65 with an insidious decline over a 10-year period.
- The average age of onset for vascular dementia is between 60 and 75. As individuals age, the risk for vascular problems (such as strokes) increases.
- Dementia with Lewy bodies typically occurs between 50 and 70 years of age.
- Frontotemporal dementia has a typical onset between 50 and 60 years of age, an earlier development than the other dementia types discussed here.

Summary of the Four Most Common Dementia Types

Condition	Symptoms	What Happens
Alzheimer's Dementia (50-75%)	Short-term memory loss	Amyloid plaques and neurofibrillary tangles
Vascular Dementia (20-30%)	Impaired executive function and attention sustainment	Large and small strokes
Dementia with Lewy Bodies (10-25%)	Visual hallucinations	Lewy body deposits on neurons
Frontotemporal Dementia (10-15%)	Personality changes	Atrophy of frontal and temporal regions of brain

Let's conclude this chapter by answering a question that is often asked: Is it possible to have a mixture of dementia subtypes? The answer is yes. In fact, approximately half of all dementias are of mixed type. For example, we can have a mix of Alzheimer's disease and vascular dementia, which occurs in approximately 15% of all cases.

With that, we're ready to jump into the next chapter where we'll discuss the risk factors for dementia.

CHAPTER TWO REFERENCES

1. Garre-Olmo J. Epidemiology of Alzheimer's disease and other dementias. *Rev Neurol.* 2018;66(11):377-386.
2. Sosa-Ortiz AL, Acosta-Castillo I, Prince MJ. Epidemiology of dementia and Alzheimer's disease. *Arch Med Res.* 2012;43(8):600-608.
3. Qiu C, De Ronchi D, Fratiglioni L. The epidemiology of the dementias: an update. *Curr Opin Psychiatry.* 2007;20(4):380-385.
4. Mayeux R, Stern Y. Epidemiology of Alzheimer disease. *Cold Spring Harb Perspect Med.* 2012;2(8):a006239-a006239. doi: 10.1101/cshperspect.a006239
5. Nichols E, Szoeke CE, Vollset SE, et al. Global, regional, and national burden of Alzheimer's disease and other dementias, 1990–2016: a systematic analysis for the Global Burden of Disease Study 2016. *Lancet Neurol.* 2019;18(1):88-106.
6. Chan KY, Wang W, Wu JJ, et al. Epidemiology of Alzheimer's disease and other forms of dementia in China, 1990–2010: a systematic review and analysis. *Lancet.* 2013;381(9882):2016-2023.
7. Corrada M, Brookmeyer R, Berlau D, Paganini-Hill A, Kawas C. Prevalence of dementia after age 90: results from the 90+ study. *Neurology.* 2008;71(5):337-343.
8. Koedam EL, Lauffer V, van der Vlies AE, van der Flier WM, Scheltens P, Pijnenburg YA. Early- versus late-onset Alzheimer's disease: More than age alone. *J Alzheimers Dis.* 2010;19(4):1401-1408.
9. Licht EA, McMurtray AM, Saul RE, Mendez MF. Cognitive differences between early-and late-onset Alzheimer's disease. *Am J Alzheimers Dis Other Demen.* 2007;22(3):218-222.
10. Cacace R, Sleegers K, Van Broeckhoven C. Molecular genetics of early-onset Alzheimer's disease revisited. *Alzheimers Dement.* 2016;12(6):733-748.
11. Tallberg I-M, Almkvist O. Confabulation and memory in patients with Alzheimer's disease. *J Clin Exp Neuropsychol.* 2001;23(2):172-184.

12. Näslund J, Schierhorn A, Hellman U, et al. Relative abundance of Alzheimer A beta amyloid peptide variants in Alzheimer disease and normal aging. *Proc Natl Acad Sci U S A*. 1994;91(18):8378-8382.
13. Shoghi-Jadid K, Small GW, Agdeppa ED, et al. Localization of neurofibrillary tangles and beta-amyloid plaques in the brains of living patients with Alzheimer disease. *Am J Geriatr Psychiatry*. 2002;10(1):24-35.
14. Pini L, Pievani M, Bocchetta M, et al. Brain atrophy in Alzheimer's disease and aging. *Ageing Res Rev*. 2016;30:25-48.
15. Liu C-C, Kanekiyo T, Xu H, Bu G. Apolipoprotein E and Alzheimer disease: risk, mechanisms and therapy. *Nat Rev Neurol*. 2013;9(2):106-118.
16. St George-Hyslop PH, Tanzi RE, Polinsky RJ, et al. The genetic defect causing familial Alzheimer's disease maps on chromosome 21. *Science*. 1987:885-890.
17. Akiyama H, Barger S, Barnum S, et al. Inflammation and Alzheimer's disease. *Neurobiol Aging*. 2000;21(3):383-421.
18. Hébert R, Brayne C. Epidemiology of vascular dementia. *Neuroepidemiology*. 1995;14(5):240-257.
19. Lis C, Gaviria M. Vascular dementia, hypertension, and the brain. *Neurol Res*. 1997;19(5):471-480.
20. Boyle PA, Cohen RA, Paul R, Moser D, Gordon N. Cognitive and motor impairments predict functional declines in patients with vascular dementia. *Int J Geriatr Psychiatry*. 2002;17(2):164-169.
21. Roh JH, Lee J-H. Recent updates on subcortical ischemic vascular dementia. *J Stroke*. 2014;16(1):18.
22. Spiegel DR, D'Souza HS, Yee K-L, et al. A case of Balint syndrome due to left basal ganglia hemorrhagic stroke: exploring the pathogenesis through parietal lobe circuits. *Prim Care Companion CNS Disord*. 2021;23(2).
23. Parvathaneni A, Das JM. Balint Syndrome. StatPearls. Updated June 27, 2022. Accessed July 6, 2022. https://www.statpearls.com/ArticleLibrary/viewarticle/18124
24. Altabakhi IW, Liang JW. Gerstmann Syndrome. StatPearls [Internet]. Updated August 29, 2022. Accessed July 11, 2022. https://www.ncbi.nlm.nih.gov/books/NBK519528/

25. Uson-Martin M, Gracia-Naya M. Top of the basilar artery syndrome: clinico-radiological aspects of 25 patients. *Rev Neurol.* 1999;28(7):698-701.
26. Smith EE. Clinical presentations and epidemiology of vascular dementia. *Clin Sci.* 2017;131(11):1059-1068.
27. Gomes J, Wachsman AM. Types of strokes. *Handbook of Clinical Nutrition and Stroke.* Springer; 2013:15-31.
28. Cirillo M, Caranci F, Tortora F, et al. Structural neuroimaging in dementia. *J Alzheimers Dis.* 2012;29(Suppl 1):16-19.
29. Price C, Jefferson A, Merino J, Heilman K, Libon D. Subcortical vascular dementia: integrating neuropsychological and neuroradiologic data. *Neurology.* 2005;65(3):376-382.
30. Garrett KD, Browndyke JN, Whelihan W, et al. The neuropsychological profile of vascular cognitive impairment—no dementia: comparisons to patients at risk for cerebrovascular disease and vascular dementia. *Arch Clin Neuropsychol.* 2004;19(6):745-757.
31. Hogan DB, Fiest KM, Roberts JI, et al. The prevalence and incidence of dementia with Lewy bodies: a systematic review. *Can J Neurol Sci.* 2016;43(S1):S83-S95.
32. Outeiro TF, Koss DJ, Erskine D, et al. Dementia with Lewy bodies: an update and outlook. *Mol Neurodegener.* 2019;14(1):1-18.
33. Bradshaw J, Saling M, Hopwood M, Anderson V, Brodtmann A. Fluctuating cognition in dementia with Lewy bodies and Alzheimer's disease is qualitatively distinct. *J Neurol Neurosurg Psychiatry.* 2004;75(3):382-387.
34. Adams D. This is Lewy Body Dementia. YouTube. September 7, 2015. Accessed December 7, 2022. https://youtu.be/oo16cWKzBbc
35. Hamdy R, Kinser A, Lewis J, et al. Hallucinations are real to patients with dementia. *Gerontol Geriatr Med.* 2017;3:2333721417721108.
36. Schenck CH, Mahowald MW. REM sleep behavior disorder: clinical, developmental, and neuroscience perspectives 16 years after its formal identification in SLEEP. *Sleep.* 2002 Mar 15;25(2):120-38. doi:10.1093/sleep/25.2.120.

37. Boeve BF. REM sleep behavior disorder: updated review of the core features, the REM sleep behavior disorder-neurodegenerative disease association, evolving concepts, controversies, and future directions. *Ann N Y Acad Sci.* 2010;1184(1):15-54.
38. Högl B, Stefani A, Videnovic A. Idiopathic REM sleep behaviour disorder and neurodegeneration—an update. *Nat Rev Neurol.* 2018;14(1):40-55.
39. Kim WS, Kågedal K, Halliday GM. Alpha-synuclein biology in Lewy body diseases. *Alzheimers Res Ther.* 2014;6(5):1-9.
40. Clinton LK, Blurton-Jones M, Myczek K, Trojanowski JQ, LaFerla FM. Synergistic interactions between Aβ, tau, and α-synuclein: acceleration of neuropathology and cognitive decline. *J Neurosci.* 2010;30(21):7281-7289.
41. Taylor J-P, Firbank MJ, He J, et al. Visual cortex in dementia with Lewy bodies: magnetic resonance imaging study. *Br J Psychiatry.* 2012;200(6):491-498.
42. Imamura T, Ishii K, Hirono N, et al. Visual hallucinations and regional cerebral metabolism in dementia with Lewy bodies (DLB). *Neuroreport.* 1999;10(9):1903-1907.
43. Jellinger KA, Korczyn AD. Are dementia with Lewy bodies and Parkinson's disease dementia the same disease? *BMC Med.* 2018;16(1):1-16.
44. Haider A, Spurling BC, Sánchez-Manso JC. Lewy Body Dementia. StatPearls [Internet]. Updated February 12, 2023. Accessed July 20, 2022. https://www.ncbi.nlm.nih.gov/books/NBK482441/
45. Urwyler P, Nef T, Müri R, et al. Visual hallucinations in eye disease and Lewy body disease. *Am J Geriatr Psychiatry.* 2016;24(5):350-358.
46. Pasquier F, Richard F, Lebert F. Natural history of frontotemporal dementia: comparison with Alzheimer's disease. *Dement Geriatr Cogn Disord.* 2004;17(4):253-257.
47. Snowden JS, Neary D, Mann DM. Frontotemporal dementia. *Br J Psychiatry.* 2002;180(2):140-143.
48. Rascovsky K, Salmon DP, Lipton A, et al. Rate of progression differs in frontotemporal dementia and Alzheimer disease. *Neurology.* 2005;65(3):397-403.

49. Marczinski CA, Davidson W, Kertesz A. A longitudinal study of behavior in frontotemporal dementia and primary progressive aphasia. *Cogn Behav Neurol.* 2004;17(4):185-190.
50. Banks SJ, Weintraub S. Neuropsychiatric symptoms in behavioral variant frontotemporal dementia and primary progressive aphasia. *J Geriatr Psychiatry Neurol.* 2008;21(2):133-141.
51. Kirshner HS. Frontotemporal dementia and primary progressive aphasia, a review. *Neuropsychiatr Dis Treat.* 2014;10:1045.
52. Paonessa F, Evans LD, Solanki R, et al. Microtubules deform the nuclear membrane and disrupt nucleocytoplasmic transport in tau-mediated frontotemporal dementia. *Cell Rep.* 2019;26(3):582-593.

PART II: **RISK FACTORS FOR DEMENTIA**

In a recent survey administered to the general population, individuals were asked to name the risk factors for dementia. The survey results revealed that a mere 1% of the general population were able to name the risk factors.[1] Even medical students struggled to provide accurate answers.[2] This may require greater attention when we consider the high prevalence of dementia among the worldwide population. Estimates indicate that at least 32% of the population will likely develop dementia.

Although none of us wants to be reminded that dementia is common, ignoring the facts can have dire consequences. One way to add a layer of protection for getting around the disease is to learn the risk factors. We should then work to minimize these risks and maximize our chances of keeping the disease at bay.

Without further ado, let's dive right into inducting ourselves into that 1% of people who can recognize the dementia risk factors.

CHAPTER THREE
THE DEMENTIA RISK FACTORS

*"Gravity has lowered my chest, my stomach, and my butt.
Why hasn't it lowered my cholesterol?"*
Randy Glasbergen

Once after presenting to a large group of individuals, an elderly lady accosted me. As if embarrassed to be overheard, she whispered, "Doctor, I have a question for you. Can sexual activity cause dementia?" I love every single question that is asked of me, and this question was no exception. Although I answered the elderly lady's question by stating that sexual activity has not been linked to dementia, there are always some exceptions to various risk factors.

As an example, rigorous sexual activity could trigger an adverse cardiovascular event, resulting in vascular-related cognitive issues. Unsanitary sexual activity could instigate a urinary tract infection, which in turn, can bring on dementia-like symptoms. As you read the dementia risk factors below, please keep in mind that there are always exceptions to each of the circumstances.

With that, let's take a look at the risk factors for dementia in no particular order of significance.

Risk Factor #1: Alcohol

Is drinking alcohol ever a good idea for the overall health of the brain? Research is conflicted. While the Mediterranean-DASH

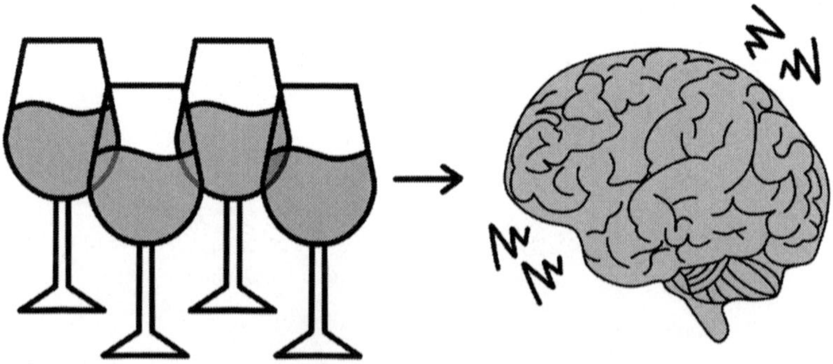

Alcohol & Cognitive Decline

Four or more drinks daily can eventually lead to cognitive decline.

Intervention for Neurodegenerative Delay (MIND) diet will be explored later in this book, that diet recommends no more than one glass of red wine daily as part of its Alzheimer's-prevention strategy. Other studies have found that drinking any alcohol may be harmful.

One thing is clear: researchers are confident that binge drinking increases susceptibility to dementia. Again, to go with the conflicted research findings theme, some studies found that even drinking moderate amounts of alcohol harms the brain's hippocampus. As discussed in the first chapter, the hippocampus is part of the brain's memory center.

In a study conducted at the University of Oxford research participants were followed for 30 years, tracking their drinking patterns and brain health. Individuals in the study who drank four or more drinks a day had 6 times the risk of hippocampus shrinkage compared to non-drinkers.[3,4]

One reason alcohol is considered harmful is due in part to alcohol's inhibitory effect on thiamine, also known as Vitamin B1, within the small intestine. Vitamin B1 helps the body absorb and generate energy from the nutrients of food. It is necessary for the growth, development, and proper functioning of the cells in the body.[5,6] Stated a different way, alcohol essentially inhibits an individual's ability to fully absorb the needed nutrients from their food. The internal cells of the body struggle with uptake of vitamin B1 or thiamine.

Insufficiencies in thiamine can lead to cerebral beriberi.[7] There are two main types of beriberi. Dry beriberi affects the nervous system, presenting as a symmetrical peripheral neuropathy. Neuropathies tend to result in numbness, tingling, muscle weakness, or pain in the affected area.[8] The second type of beriberi is known as wet beriberi and is associated with cardiovascular problems.[9,10]

We can't talk about thiamine deficiencies without also mentioning Wernicke-Korsakoff syndrome. The deficiencies in Wernicke-Korsakoff includes gait changes, prominent impairment in memory formation (anterograde amnesia), and eye movement abnormalities.[11] The confusion and loss of muscle coordination symptoms has been ascribed to damage to the thalamus and hypothalamus regions of the brain. It is essential that intravenous (IV) thiamine is administered as soon as possible to prevent further damage to the central nervous system.

Other Risk Factors Associated with Alcohol. The potential for prescription drug and alcohol interaction side effects cannot be ignored. Unfortunately, the mixing of prescription drugs and alcohol is much more common than one might expect. One study found that at least 63% of older adults admitted to simultaneous use of prescription medications and alcohol.[12] Even interactions involving nonprescription medications (eg, aspirin, vitamins) can be significant. In addition to acting as an inhibitor of thiamine, alcohol tends to act as an inhibitor on several enzyme systems in the liver. Inhibition of enzyme systems can increase a drug to toxic or lethal levels.[13]

On the other hand, chronic alcohol use results in liver damage, which can act as an inducer of enzyme systems.[14] Inducers of enzyme systems result in decreased levels of a drug. Individuals with multiple health conditions such as diabetes, hypertension, and depression may have the most significant adverse interactions, which can result in cognitive impairment that may resemble a dementia condition.

As previously mentioned, some studies have indicated that any alcohol use is considered harmful. In other words, there is no amount of liquor, wine, or beer that is safe for overall health. In one study conducted at the University of Oxford, the relationship between self-reported alcohol intake of approximately 25,000 people in the United Kingdom and their brain scans was examined. Findings showed that drinking had a detrimental effect on the gray matter of the brain. The more an individual consumed alcohol, the lower volume of gray matter found.[4]

As you might recall, gray matter is the thinking part of the brain where information is processed. The less gray matter an individual has, the worse the outcome on memory exams. Although alcohol made only a small contribution to decreasing gray matter in the brain (0.8%), it was a greater contribution than other modifiable risk factors.[4] Modifiable risk factors are things we can do something about. This is in contrast to non-modifiable risk factors (eg, aging or genetics).

It is also notable that the study cited above also found that it did not matter what type of alcoholic beverage was consumed. Whether the alcohol consists of wine, spirits or beer, the mere content of alcohol in the drink is a debilitating factor on the brain. Having certain characteristics, such as hypertension or obesity can put individuals at higher risk for adverse effects on the brain.

The adverse effects of alcohol on the brain appear to present with subtle changes that may not be immediately apparent during routine neuropsychological examinations. Over time, there may be more obvious changes associated with weakened memory.

Risk Factor #2: Genetics

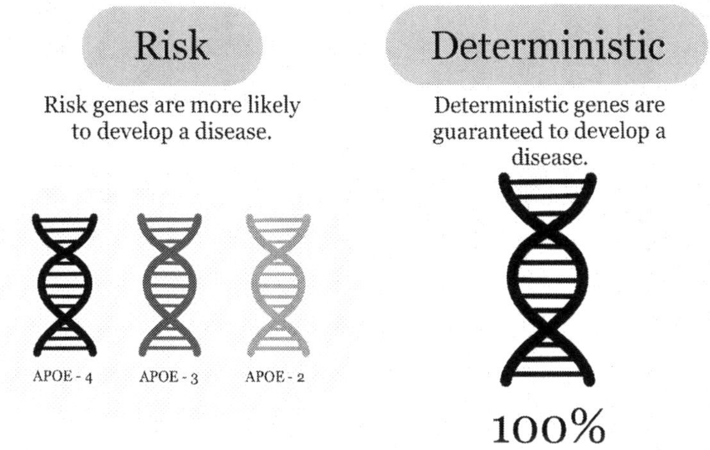

Research indicates that some forms of Alzheimer's disease may run in families. As you might recall, beta-amyloid is produced by mutations of chromosome 21, akin to what is seen with Down syndrome. It is the specific mutations of chromosome 21 that appears to produce familial Alzheimer's disease.[15]

Although a family history of Alzheimer's is not necessary for an individual to develop the disease, having a parent or sibling with Alzheimer's increases the risk of developing the disease. This is in contrast to individuals who do not have a first-degree relative with Alzheimer's.[16] In fact, those who have more than one first-degree relative with Alzheimer's are at an even higher risk for neurodegenerative disease.

Alzheimer's disease associated with the genetic type tends to have an earlier age of onset compared to individuals with the non-genetic type. The genetic type of onset usually occurs prior to age 65 (between age 30-60). Individuals with the non-genetic type of Alzheimer's tend to have an onset at approximately 65 years of age (categorized as a "late onset" type).[17] Interestingly, some studies have shown that early onset Alzheimer's type tends to have a more rapid progression of symptoms compared to later onset type.[18-20]

When discussing the risks associated with genetics, there are two categories of genes that influence whether a person develops a disease: risk genes and deterministic genes. Researchers have identified Alzheimer's genes in both categories. Let's explore the differences between the two categories.

Risk Genes. As its name implies, risk genes are associated with an increased likelihood of developing a disease.[21] However, risk genes do not guarantee that a disease will happen. Several genes that increase the risk of Alzheimer's have been found. From the readings in the previous chapter, you know one risk gene as the apolipoprotein E-e4 (APOE-e4). APOE-e4 is found on chromosome 19 and is the first risk gene identified for Alzheimer's. It remains the gene with the strongest impact on risk for the disease.[22]

Deterministic Genes. Deterministic genes directly cause a disease. With a deterministic gene, you are basically guaranteed to develop a given disease. In the case of Alzheimer's, deterministic genes are, fortunately, rare. How rare? Deterministic genes for Alzheimer's have been found in only a few hundred extended families worldwide.[23]

The differences between risk genes and deterministic genes are summarized in the illustration on the previous page. Recall that the neurotransmitter, acetylcholine, plays a role in memory functions. Individuals with a deterministic gene may produce lower than normal acetylcholine levels, which can have a negative effect on memory functions.

What About the Genetics Associated with Ethnicity?

Prior research findings indicate that ethnicity plays a role in the risk for dementia, with some groups being at higher risk. Based on the research published in 2016, African Americans have the highest risk of dementia with a 38% increase over a 25-year period beginning at age 65. African Americans are followed by American Indian/Alaska Natives at 35%. Latinos are the next group at 32% with Whites at 30%. The two ethnicities with the lowest risks are Asian Americans at 28% and Pacific Islanders at 25%.[24]

Differences among ethnicities for dementia risk have been ascribed to factors such as higher prevalence of hypertension (high blood pressure) and diabetes compared to other ethnic groups with lower risks.[25,26]

Risk Factor #3: Smoking

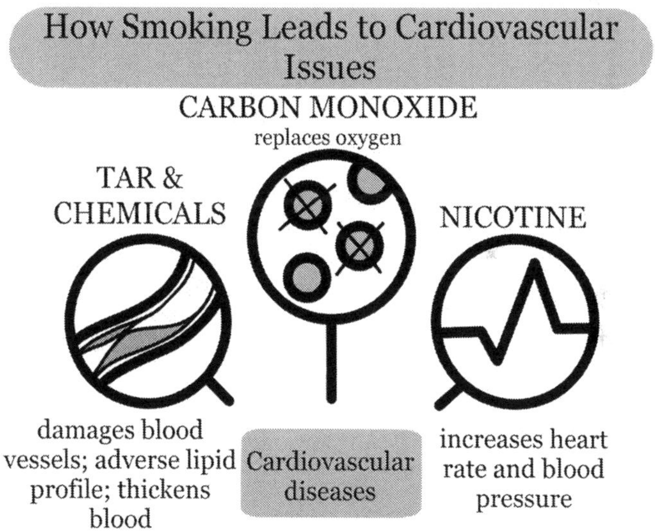

Although most everyone and their dog knows that smoking is bad for your health, let me give you another reason to quit. Giving up smoking could lower your risk for developing dementia.[27-30]

The nicotine in cigarettes and other tobacco products causes blood vessels to become narrower. Heart rate also increases. The combination of the narrowing of blood vessels and increased heart rate leads to an approximately 6% increase in blood pressure from smoking a single cigarette.[31] Imagine what smoking multiple cigarettes can do to blood pressure.

Since heightened blood pressure also affects the risk for vascular disease, it follows that smoking increases the risk for vascular dementia.[32,33] If the aforementioned reasons are not enough to convince you to quit smoking, here's more good news: hope is not lost no matter how long an individual has smoked. As soon as a person quits smoking, the risk for dementia decreases.[34]

Risk Factor #4: High Blood Pressure

The National Health and Nutrition Examination Survey study found that, unfortunately, only one-half of Americans with hypertension (HTN) had adequate blood pressure control.[35] Blood pressure measures the force applied to your arteries. The arteries are blood vessels that carry blood circulated from the heart to our

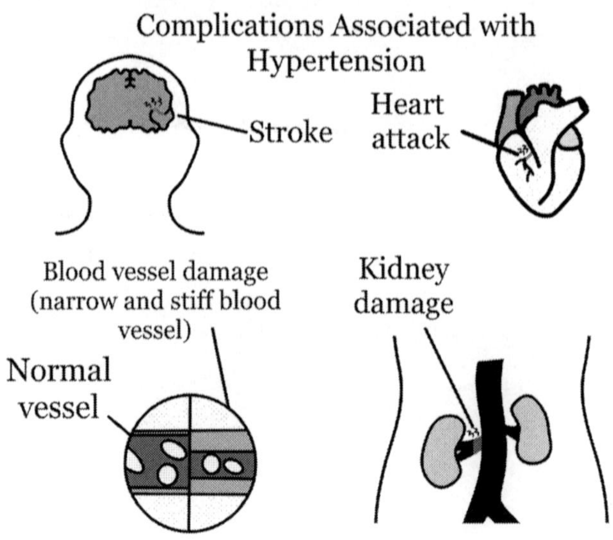

essential organs (brain, kidneys, liver, and lungs). Blood pressure can be taken from several places on the body, including the biceps, wrist, thigh, or ankle.

Your blood pressure is reported as two numbers. The first or top number represents the systolic pressure. Systolic pressure measures the pressure on your arteries per beat of the heart. In the second or bottom number, diastolic pressure indicates the remaining pressure when the heart rests between beats.

A healthy blood pressure reading is dependent on several factors involving age, body mass, and weight.[36,37] Generally speaking, a normal blood pressure reading is below 120/80 mm Hg (millimeters of mercury). High blood pressure or hypertension (HTN) is diagnosed when your blood pressure is consistently above the aforementioned range (especially at 130/80 or 140/90 mm Hg).[38-40] Aiming to maintain a systolic (top number) blood pressure of 130 mm Hg or less in midlife—from around 40 years of age—is a good goal for maintaining optimal cognitive and overall health. Making lifestyle modifications such as healthier food choices and consistent exercise are strongly encouraged to maintain a < 130 mm Hg blood pressure reading.

In addition to lifestyle modifications, medications to lower blood pressure (ie, antihypertensives) are strongly recommended. In fact, it has been said that antihypertensive medications are the only known effective preventative medication for dementia![41]

It is important to recognize that HTN is a serious condition. Individuals with HTN are much more likely to have a heart attack or stroke.[42,43] Long term HTN damages blood vessels in the kidney, heart, and brain. Moreover, individuals with HTN are more likely to develop vascular dementia.[44]

In addition to HTN's propensity to increase the risk for stroke or heart disease, HTN has been found to be associated with greater brain shrinkage.[45] Those without HTN or who engaged in intensive cognitive activity were found to limit the effect of overall brain shrinkage, particularly for the cerebellum (which can have implications for motor control and postural adjustments to maintain balance). We will further discuss blood pressure monitoring and cognitive training as dementia prevention measures in Chapter 5.

Risk Factor #5: Depression

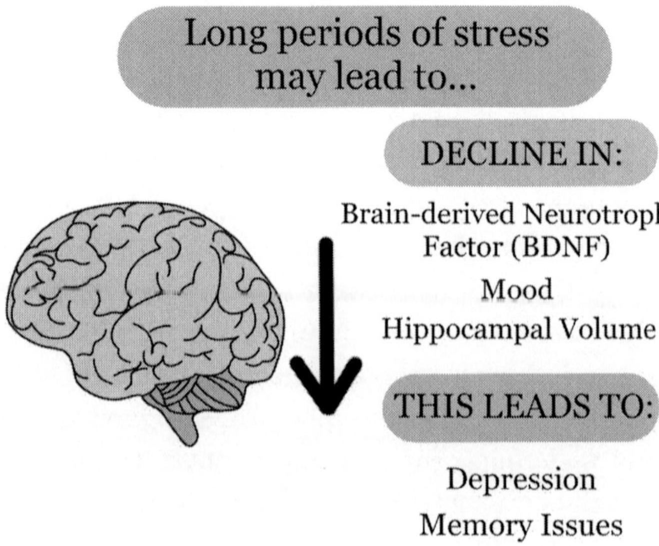

You may be surprised to learn that depression is considered a risk factor. Research has found that individuals with untreated depression symptoms have a 35% faster rate of cognitive decline than those with no depression symptoms.[46-48]

Symptoms of hopelessness, loss of interest in activities, energy, sleep, or concentration are all indicators that there may be something wrong with the brain. It is important to note that individuals with depression often have struggles with learning and memory functions, which can mimic dementia symptoms.[49] Moreover, individuals with dementia often present with depression symptoms.[50] This can make it difficult to differentiate whether someone is struggling from depression or dementia, creating barriers to obtaining effective treatment.

It is important to recognize that depression tends to manifest differently in older adults compared to younger adults. There are fewer "typical" symptoms of sadness, blue mood, and tearfulness. Rather, in older adults, there may be withdrawal from social events, energy loss, and bodily symptoms associated with pain, low appetite, or insomnia.[51] It is easy to overlook or miss these less typical symptoms in older adults.

Neuropsychological exams are especially helpful in parsing out depression from dementia as well as other potential healthcare issues.[52,53] Examples of other potential healthcare issues that neuropsychological exams can clarify and assist with diagnostic differentiation include chronic stress, diabetes, or thyroid problems. Once appropriately diagnosed, neuropsychological exams can provide appropriate recommendations to treat the symptoms in order to improve cognitive issues.

How does depression lead to increased risk for dementia development? Research has shown that depression can create an unhealthy environment within the brain. Consider, for example, stress. Stress can contribute to reduction of glucocorticoids in the brain and body. Glucocorticoids are a beneficial hormone that helps with keeping the body healthy, such as controlling how your cells use sugar and fat. Glucocorticoids also help curb inflammation.[54]

As glucocorticoids are diminished, the inflammation creates conditions in which neurons become subject to atrophy and eventual apoptosis (cell death). Reduced glucocorticoids create an environment that isn't conducive to something called brain-derived neurotrophic factor (BDNF).[55] You may be aware that BDNF is a peptide—or long-chain protein—that benefits the brain by acting as a growth factor for the brain's neurons.

Think of BDNF as fertilizer for the brain. Just as we might use fertilize on our garden rose bushes to maximize the bloom, BDNF can be compared to fertilizer for the brain's neurons. It is important to remember, though, that it is not just fertilizer that we need to maximize the potential of our rose bushes. We also need to prune and water the rose bushes and protect them from droughts and heat waves.

In the same way, it is not just BDNF that we need for our brains. The pruning of our rose bushes might represent limiting the potentially harmful effects of chronic stress with good coping skills.

Watering of our rose bushes along with measures to protect them from droughts and heat waves can be represented by ensuring that we address our healthcare needs by engaging in self-care practices (eg, attending annual physicals or other healthcare services, practicing good dental hygiene, getting enough sleep, eating balanced meals, and engaging in a consistent exercise routine).

The point here is that depression usually means that our brains are not functioning optimally. When the brain does not function optimally, it can become more vulnerable to dementia. Depression essentially impairs the brain's ability to engage in BDNF driven neurogenesis. This impairment leads to a decrease in hippocampal volume, as determined by magnetic resonance imaging in depressed patients.[56] Decreases in hippocampal volume leads to memory problems. These decreases in hippocampal volume are also seen in individuals with post-traumatic stress disorder or other mental health states in which there is significant release of stress-induced cortisol in the brain.

This is why it is important to get help for depression or other negative mental health states. Don't let your mental health go without care, not when there is help available.

A common question is if there is a link between hearing loss and depression. The link between hearing loss and depression is interesting, particularly among individuals with late onset hearing loss. Consider, for example, an individual who is thrown a birthday party by a loved one. Although a birthday party should be an enjoyable event with opportunities to socialize with friends and loved ones, some individuals may be unhappy because they may think that they are not really the center of attention (for the lack of a better phrase). The individual may feel that people are just talking around or about them. They may also not understand that these commentaries are only part of regular conversation.

For individuals who do not rely on a visual means for communication (such as a signed language) or who have late-onset hearing loss, they may rely on vocal auditory methods. Use of vocal auditory methods includes use of hearing aids or cochlear implants. The use of these hearing assistive devices may give these individuals the ability to continue to engage in conversation with family members and friends. Since we are social creatures, connection with others as part of a balanced lifestyle can help buffer stress and ward off symptoms of depression. Sometimes addressing hearing with non-pharmacological methods can have indirect benefits to cognitive function and overall health.

I remember an individual sharing a story about a social gathering. As the lone individual with hearing loss at the gathering, he shared the difficulties that night of trying to join in conversations among the hearing individuals. Due to the fast-paced nature of the conversations as well as background noise that obscured communication, it was difficult to engage with any one person, let alone the small, congregated groups.

The reason this story stuck with me is because of what happened at the gathering. The individual perceived the hearing associates around him as talking about him. Already feeling socially isolated, this individual lashed out in a tragic physical confrontation toward several hearing individuals. Lack of access to social communication can have a powerful influence on one's mood and behaviors.

Risk Factor #6: Diabetes

Diabetes is a condition that affects how your body turns food into energy. When we eat, most of the food is broken down into sugar (also known as glucose). The glucose is released into the bloodstream. When glucose increases following a meal, it signals to the pancreas to release insulin. Insulin can be thought of as a key that opens the door to the body's cells, allowing glucose into the cell to use as energy.[57]

If someone has been diagnosed with diabetes, they may not have enough insulin "keys" to open the doors to the body's cells to

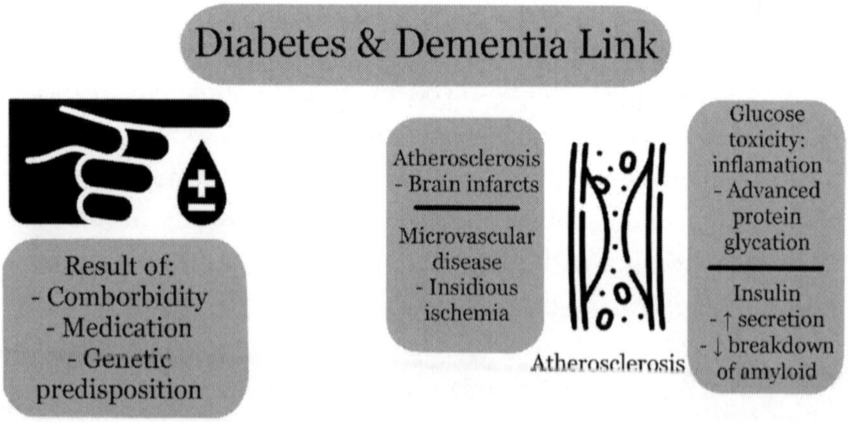

allow glucose inside to generate energy. At other times, the insulin keys may be broken, rendering the insulin ineffective at opening the door to the body's cells. When there isn't enough insulin to allow glucose inside the body's cells, too much glucose stays in the bloodstream, creating harmful repercussions for the body's organs.

Diabetes can be broken down into Type 1 and Type 2 (gestational diabetes can also be considered a third type of diabetes but won't be covered here). Type 1 diabetes was formerly recognized as juvenile-onset or insulin-dependent diabetes. Think of Type 1 diabetes as essentially not having a key (insulin), or enough keys, to open the body's cell doors.

With Type 1 diabetes, there appears to be an autoimmune reaction in which the body attacks itself by mistake, effectively stopping the body from making insulin. Approximately 5-10% of people with diabetes have Type 1, which is usually diagnosed in children, teens, and young adults.[58] Insulin must be taken on a daily basis in Type 1 diabetes. There are no known prevention strategies for Type 1 diabetes.

Individuals with Type 2 diabetes don't respond to insulin as well as they should.[59] Later in the disease, they often do not make enough insulin. Individuals with Type 2 diabetes can be thought of as having a broken key. When there are one too many broken keys (or ineffective insulin), glucose cannot get inside the cells. Blood sugar then rises above normal levels. Around 90-95% of people with diabetes have Type 2.[58]

Type 2 diabetes tends to develop over the years and is usually diagnosed in adults. However, more and more children and teens are being diagnosed. Type 2 diabetes can be helped or delayed with a healthy lifestyle (eg, losing weight, exercising, eating sensibly).

How Diabetes Increases Dementia Risk. Current research suggests that individuals with diabetes have approximately 75% higher risk of dementia. The causative factors appear to relate to hyperglycemia (high blood sugar or glucose), which causes inflammation inside of the body.[60,61] Chronic inflammation can damage brain cells and trigger a cascading effect that leads to problems with cognition. Given the vascular inflammation in the human body, heart disease and stroke are another risk factor associated with diabetes.[62,63]

Damaged blood vessels in the brain can contribute to a dementia condition. The problems associated with hyperglycemia appears to be most elevated for Type 2 diabetes.[64] In fact, heart disease and stroke are twice as common in those with Type 2 diabetes compared to the nondiabetic population.[65] Diabetic women are also more vulnerable to vascular disease compared to diabetic men.[66]

The elephant in the room now becomes the question of whether people with Type 1 diabetes are also considered a dementia risk factor. Unfortunately, this is a new area of research for which we are still gathering information. The few published studies seem to suggest that individuals with poorly controlled Type 1 diabetes with multiple episodes of hypoglycemic and hyperglycemic events over the long term may have increased dementia risk.[67,68]

We also know that individuals with Type 1 diabetes must be vigilant concerning maintenance of insulin levels. For many years, it was generally considered that the brain was insensitive to insulin. It is now accepted that insulin has central neuromodulatory functions.[69,70] The fluctuations with insulin control may invite times that the brain becomes unbalanced with too little or too much insulin. Such non-optimal levels of insulin may potentially trigger a cascade of neurochemical factors that potentially increase dementia risk.

The Hearing Loss & Diabetes Connection. You may be interested to know that hearing loss in a person with diabetes often presents earlier than in those without diabetes.[71] The risk for hearing loss in a person with diabetes increases when there are co-conditions, such as neuropathies, high blood pressure, and cardiovascular disease.

The hearing loss and diabetes connection is not surprising when one considers the damage that elevated blood glucose has on the small vessels in the human body. Higher levels of blood glucose can damage the smaller vessels in the inner ear and disrupt normal hearing.[71] The severity of the hearing loss depends on the

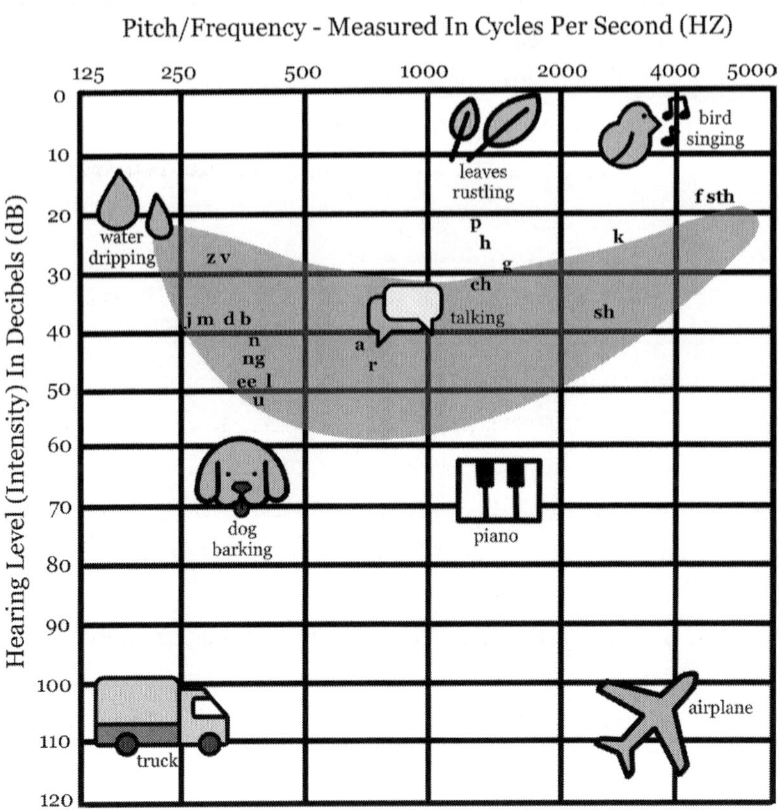

extent of the damage to the vessels of the inner ear. The illustration below shows an audiogram with sample sounds that show what an individual with hearing loss may or may not hear.

Risk Factor #7: Social Isolation

Although social isolation is a common experience for many, it is especially prevalent in our deaf and hard of hearing population. In my clinical practice, I frequently see deaf, hard of hearing, and deafblind individuals who experience significant social isolation in their lives. One patient, who we'll refer to as John, is an extreme and tragic example. John was placed in a group home setting in his mid-30s. His primary and preferred communication modality was American Sign Language (ASL). The problem with the group home placement was that none of the staff members was ASL-fluent.

Fast forward to more than 30 years later. When a change in John's guardianship occurred, the guardian immediately recognized the gravity of the situation. The guardian sought me out and brought John in for weekly therapy sessions. John had been living in the group home for more than three decades with essentially minimal exposure to a reliable language. Although previously fluent in ASL, John's language skills were markedly deteriorated when I met him. He was also heavily sedated with antipsychotic medications.

As I learned more about John's medical history, it became apparent that antipsychotics were used following increased agitation over the years in the group home. This begs the question: Who would not become agitated—potentially to the point of physical aggression—if deprived of language stimulation or opportunities to socialize with others?

Further perpetuating feelings of isolation for people whose primary language is a signed language are those with family members or neighbors who may not sign. Research indicates that about 95% of children with hearing loss are born to parents with normal hearing (the rest are born to deaf parents).[73]

Of the deaf children born to hearing parents, very few have parents or siblings who can sign. Estimates indicate that only approximately 25% of hearing parents can sign fluently. If we consider any kind of signing—regardless of fluency—the best estimate is 40% of families use some form of signing at home.[74] The lack of access to individuals who can sign can exacerbate social isolation or feelings of loneliness.

Research has shown that social isolation—even the perception of it—can have serious negative effects on both physical and mental health. Individuals who are lonely or isolated are more likely to have heart disease, stroke, or a weakened immune system.[75-78] Experiencing loneliness, especially chronic loneliness, may also aggravate other health problems, including recovery from serious health conditions such as cancer.[79,80]

Social isolation can also be stressful. Increased blood pressure (hypertension) via stress-induced release of norepinephrine in the brain has been found in individuals experiencing symptoms of loneliness.[81] It is also clear that loneliness is closely linked to depression and obesity.[82] All of these negative factors can lead to an early death.

It should be noted that individuals with late-onset hearing loss may be at higher risk for social isolation than individuals who are part of the deaf community. The higher risk for individuals with late-onset hearing loss can be ascribed to a personal decision to withdraw from prior social activities and connections due to the increased communication difficulties brought on by the hearing loss. Although there is a subset of individuals who are culturally Deaf and use ASL who may also be socially isolated, a significant number have strong social connections within this community. The protective factor of these deaf communities in terms of maintaining social connections will be explored further in Chapter 5.

Mixed Dementia and Other Contributory Risk Factors

A question that I am often asked is if it's possible to have a mixture of dementia subtypes. The answer is yes. Half of all dementia cases are a single type of dementia, such as Alzheimer's, vascular, or Lewy body. The other half is of a mixed nature, meaning that they are a combination of two or more types of dementia. For example, we can have a mix of Alzheimer's disease and vascular dementia, which occurs in approximately 15% of all cases.

It is important to remember that while the aforementioned risk factors have been determined by research to be associated with increased risk for dementia onset, there are a number of other factors that can exacerbate risk for one of the dementia subtypes. For example, individuals who have sustained a traumatic brain injury (TBI) have an exacerbated risk for Alzheimer's if they also have one of the aforementioned seven risk factors[83]. The eighth risk factor will be discussed in the next chapter.

Access to minimal or lower education levels during early life is also considered an exacerbating risk factor. Lower education levels are thought to be associated with a lower cognitive reserve and is considered an early life risk (younger than 45 years). Research support for less education being an exacerbating risk factor includes previous findings of increased connectivity in the temporal and frontal brain areas for individuals who have exposure to cognitive stimulation in the classroom or otherwise.[84-86]

Individuals with hearing loss who may not have had language stimulation during the critical period of development (birth to five years of age) frequently face lifelong communication difficulties.[87-89] Problems with communication are often associated with receptive comprehension skills. As one can imagine, without strong receptive comprehension skills, it can make learning and education extremely difficult to attain. Even within an Ivy League academic setting, language barriers essentially relegate a high-quality institution into an impoverished educational environment.

For those with hearing loss, language deprivation can be an exacerbating risk factor.

Other exacerbating risk factors include hyperlipidemia (high cholesterol) and obesity.[90,91] These exacerbating factors can be considered part of the vascular risk factors that include the aforementioned risks associated with hypertension and diabetes. As we know, vascular risk factors are frequently associated with a sedentary lifestyle. Further substantiating this finding is the fact that several long-term studies have shown exercise to be associated with a reduced risk of dementia (discussed in Chapter 5).

Secondhand smoke is another example of an exacerbating risk factor. Vulnerability to dementia risk is also increased the more one is exposed to poor air quality or air pollution.

Finally, we would not do this chapter justice without mentioning one last contributory risk factor: post-traumatic stress disorder (PTSD). PTSD has also been found to be associated with an approximately twofold increased risk of dementia.[92] Interestingly, the same study found that combat veterans with PTSD have a lower dementia risk compared with their counterparts with the disorder from the general population.

The lower dementia risk may be associated with the fact that veterans are typically more likely to receive treatment for PTSD. These findings suggest that treating PTSD may potentially reduce subsequent dementia risk. PTSD seems to accelerate cognitive decline through what has been described as a "wearing down" effect on the brain, brought on by continuous stress and subsequent vulnerability to dementia.

Note that, given the COVID-19 pandemic, individuals hospitalized with COVID-19 can be at risk for PTSD. This is especially significant if the individual experienced or even witnessed a severe life-threatening infection. It may be prudent to pursue follow-up and screening for PTSD for these individuals.

Key Takeaways

Congratulations! You have just been inducted into the 1% of people who are aware of the main risk factors for dementia. Let's review the seven risk factors for dementia:

- **Risk Factor #1: Alcohol**. Excess alcohol consumption increases susceptibility to dementia.
- **Risk Factor #2: Smoking**. As soon as a person quits smoking, the risk for dementia decreases.
- **Risk Factor #3: Genetics**. Having more than one first-degree relative with dementia is an elevating risk factor.
- **Risk Factor #4: High Blood Pressure**. Individuals with hypertension are more likely to have a stroke, which increases the risk for dementia, particularly vascular dementia.
- **Risk Factor #5: Depression**. Individuals with untreated depression symptoms have a 35% faster cognitive decline than those with no depression.
- **Risk Factor #6: Diabetes**. High blood sugar causes inflammation inside the body, which can increase the risk for brain cell damage and trigger a cascading effect that leads to problems with cognition.
- **Risk Factor #7: Social Isolation**. Individuals who are lonely or isolated are not only at increased risk for dementia onset but are more likely to have heart disease, stroke, or a longer time to recover from a healthcare condition.

The eighth risk factor is one that is unique to most reading this book: hearing loss. It is to this risk we turn to in Part Three.

CHAPTER THREE REFERENCES

1. Stevens J, Philp N, Phipps L, Fossey I. *Dementia Attitudes Monitor*. Alzheimer's Research UK;2018.
2. Morgan J, Bindoff A, Doherty K, Vickers J, Alty J. Are tomorrow's doctors prepared to prevent dementia? A cross-sectional study of Tasmanian medical students' knowledge of dementia risk factors. *J Clin Neurosci*. 2022;96:133-137. doi: 10.1016/j.jocn.2021.11.005
3. Topiwala A, Allan CL, Valkanova V, et al. Moderate alcohol consumption as risk factor for adverse brain outcomes and cognitive decline: longitudinal cohort study. *BMJ*. 2017;357.
4. Topiwala A, Ebmeier KP, Maullin-Sapey T, Nichols TE. Alcohol consumption and MRI markers of brain structure and function: cohort study of 25,378 UK Biobank participants. *NeuroImage Clin*. 2022;35:103066. doi: 10.1016/j.nicl.2022.103066
5. Gibson GE, Hirsch JA, Fonzetti P, Jordon BD, Cirio RT, Elder J. Vitamin B1 (thiamine) and dementia. *Ann N Y Acad Sci*. 2016;1367(1):21.
6. Fattal-Valevski A. Thiamine (vitamin B1). *J Evid Based Complementary Altern Med*. 2011;16(1):12-20.
7. Wiley KD, Gupta M. Vitamin B1 Thiamine deficiency. StatPearls [Internet]. Updated July 22, 2022. Accessed July 21, 2022. https://www.ncbi.nlm.nih.gov/books/NBK537204/
8. Martyn C, Hughes R. Epidemiology of peripheral neuropathy. neurology Neurol, *Neurosurg Psychiatry*. 1997;62(4):310.
9. Chisolm-Straker M, Cherkas D. Altered and unstable: wet beriberi, a clinical review. *J Emerg Med*. 2013 Sep;45(3):341-344. doi:10.1016/j.jemermed.2013.04.022
10. DiNicolantonio JJ, Liu J, O'Keefe JH. Thiamine and cardiovascular disease: a literature review. *Prog Cardiovasc Dis*. 2018;61(1):27-32.
11. Isenberg-Grzeda E, Kutner HE, Nicolson SE. Wernicke-Korsakoff syndrome: under-recognized and under-treated. *Psychosomatics*. 2012;53(6):507-516.
12. Immonen S, Valvanne J, Pitkälä KH. The prevalence of potential alcohol–drug interactions in older adults. *Scand J Prim Health Care*. 2013;31(2):73-78.

13. Alatalo PI, Koivisto HM, Hietala JP, Puukka KS, Bloigu R, Niemelä OJ. Effect of moderate alcohol consumption on liver enzymes increases with increasing body mass index. *Am J Clin Nutr.* 2008;88(4):1097-1103.
14. Lieber CS. Relationships between nutrition, alcohol use, and liver disease. *Alcohol Res.* 2003;27(3):220.
15. St George-Hyslop PH, Tanzi RE, Polinsky RJ, et al. The genetic defect causing familial Alzheimer's disease maps on chromosome 21. *Science.* 1987:885-890.
16. Mayeux R, Sano M, Chen J, Tatemichi T, Stern Y. Risk of dementia in first-degree relatives of patients with Alzheimer's disease and related disorders. *Arch Neurol.* 1991;48(3):269-273.
17. Chiaravalloti A, Koch G, Toniolo S, et al. Comparison between early-onset and late-onset Alzheimer's disease patients with amnestic presentation: CSF and 18F-FDG PET study. *Dement Geriatr Cogn Dis Extra.* 2016;6(1):108-119. doi: 10.1159/000441776
18. Jacobs D, Sano M, Marder K, et al. Age at onset of Alzheimer's disease: relation to pattern of cognitive dysfunction and rate of decline. *Neurology.* 1994;44(7):1215-1215.
19. Toyota Y, Ikeda M, Shinagawa S, et al. Comparison of behavioral and psychological symptoms in early-onset and late-onset Alzheimer's disease. *Int J Geriatr Psychiatry.* 2007;22(9):896-901. doi: 10.1002/gps.1760
20. Kim EJ, Cho SS, Jeong Y, et al. Glucose metabolism in early onset versus late onset Alzheimer's disease: an SPM analysis of 120 patients. *Brain.* 2005;128(8):1790-1801. doi: 10.1093/brain/awh539
21. Chao S, Roberts JS, Marteau TM, Silliman R, Cupples LA, Green RC. Health behavior changes after genetic risk assessment for Alzheimer disease: The REVEAL Study. *Alzheimer Dis Assoc Disord.* 2008;22(1):94.
22. Coon KD, Myers AJ, Craig DW, et al. A high-density whole-genome association study reveals that APOE is the major susceptibility gene for sporadic late-onset Alzheimer's disease. *J Clin Psychiatry.* 2007;68(4):8183.

23. Williamson J, Goldman J, Marder KS. Genetic aspects of Alzheimer disease. *Neurologist.* 2009;15(2):80.
24. Mayeda ER, Glymour MM, Quesenberry CP, Whitmer RA. Inequalities in dementia incidence between six racial and ethnic groups over 14 years. *Alzheimers Dement.* 2016;12(3):216-224.
25. Mayeda ER, Karter AJ, Huang ES, Moffet HH, Haan MN, Whitmer RA. Racial/ethnic differences in dementia risk among older type 2 diabetic patients: the diabetes and aging study. *Diabetes Care.* 2014;37(4):1009-1015.
26. Chen C, Zissimopoulos JM. Racial and ethnic differences in trends in dementia prevalence and risk factors in the United States. *Alzheimers Dement (N Y).* 2018;4:510-520.
27. Zhong G, Wang Y, Zhang Y, Guo JJ, Zhao Y. Smoking is associated with an increased risk of dementia: a meta-analysis of prospective cohort studies with investigation of potential effect modifiers. *PLoS One.* 2015;10(3):e0118333.
28. Peters R, Poulter R, Warner J, Beckett N, Burch L, Bulpitt C. Smoking, dementia and cognitive decline in the elderly, a systematic review. *BMC Geriatr.* 2008;8(1):1-7.
29. Anstey KJ, von Sanden C, Salim A, O'Kearney R. Smoking as a risk factor for dementia and cognitive decline: a meta-analysis of prospective studies. *Am J Epidemiol.* 2007;166(4):367-378.
30. Choi D, Choi S, Park SM. Effect of smoking cessation on the risk of dementia: a longitudinal study. *Ann Clin Transl Neurol.* 2018;5(10):1192-1199.
31. Kool MJ, Hoeks AP, Boudier HAS, Reneman RS, Van Bortel LM. Short and long-term effects of smoking on arterial wall properties in habitual smokers. *J Am Coll Cardiol.* 1993;22(7):1881-1886.
32. Román GC. Vascular dementia prevention: a risk factor analysis. *Cerebrovasc Dis.* 2005;20(Suppl. 2):91-100.
33. Hasnain M, Vieweg VR. Possible role of vascular risk factors in Alzheimer's disease and vascular dementia. *Curr Pharm Des.* 2014;20(38):6007-6013.
34. Lu Y, Sugawara Y, Zhang S, Tomata Y, Tsuji I. Smoking cessation and incident dementia in elderly Japanese: the Ohsaki Cohort 2006 Study. *Eur J Epidemiol.* 2020:1-10.

35. Nwankwo T, Yoon SS, Burt VL, Gu Q. Hypertension among adults in the United States: national health and nutrition examination survey, 2011-2012. *NCHS Data Brief.* 2013; Oct(133):1-8.
36. Pickering TG, Hall JE, Appel LJ, et al. Recommendations for blood pressure measurement in humans and experimental animals: part 1: blood pressure measurement in humans: a statement for professionals from the Subcommittee of Professional and Public Education of the American Heart Association Council on High Blood Pressure Research. *Circulation.* 2005;111(5):697-716. doi: 10.1161/01.CIR.0000154900.76284.F6
37. Beevers G, Lip GY, O'Brien E. Blood pressure measurement: Part I—Sphygmomanometry: Factors common to all techniques. *BMJ.* 2001;322(7292):981-985.
38. Wermelt J, Schunkert H. Management of arterial hypertension. *Herz.* 2017;42(5):515-526.
39. Jordan J, Kurschat C, Reuter H. Arterial hypertension: diagnosis and treatment. *Deutsches Ärzteblatt International.* 2018;115(33-34):557.
40. Jarvis C. *Physical Examination and Health Assessment.* 8th ed. Elsevier Health Sciences; 2018.
41. Livingston G, Huntley J, Sommerlad A, et al. Dementia prevention, intervention, and care: 2020 report of the Lancet Commission. *Lancet.* 2020;396(10248):413-446. doi: 10.1016/s0140-6736(20)30367-6
42. Wajngarten M, Silva GS. Hypertension and stroke: update on treatment. *Eur Cardiol.* 2019;14(2):111.
43. Johansson BB. Hypertension mechanisms causing stroke. *Clin Exp Pharmacol Physiol.* 1999;26(7):563-565.
44. Sharp SI, Aarsland D, Day S, Sønnesyn H, Group AsSVDSR, Ballard C. Hypertension is a potential risk factor for vascular dementia: systematic review. *Int J Geriatr Psychiatry.* 2011;26(7):661-669.
45. Raz N, Schmiedek F, Rodrigue KM, Kennedy KM, Lindenberger U, Lövdén M. Differential brain shrinkage over 6 months shows limited association with cognitive practice. *Brain Cogn.* 2013;82(2):171-180.

46. Wilson RS, Mendes de Leon CF, Bennett DA, Bienias JL, Evans DA. Depressive symptoms and cognitive decline in a community population of older persons. *J Neurol Neurosurg Psychiatry.* 2004;75(1):126-129. https://jnnp.bmj.com/content/jnnp/75/1/126.full.pdf
47. Wilson RS, Capuano AW, Boyle PA, et al. Clinical-pathologic study of depressive symptoms and cognitive decline in old age. *Neurology.* 2014;83(8):702-709.
48. Zheng F, Zhong B, Song X, Xie W. Persistent depressive symptoms and cognitive decline in older adults. *Br J Psychiatry.* 2018;213(5):638-644.
49. Fischer P. The spectrum of depressive pseudo-dementia. In: Jellinger KA, Windich M, eds. *New Trends in the Diagnosis and Therapy of Non-Alzheimer's Dementia.* Springer; 1996:193-203.
50. Enache D, Winblad B, Aarsland D. Depression in dementia: epidemiology, mechanisms, and treatment. *Curr Opin Psychiatry.* 2011;24(6):461-472.
51. Fiske A, Wetherell JL, Gatz M. Depression in older adults. *Ann Rev Clin Psychiatry.* 2009;5:363-389. doi: 10.1146/annurev.clinpsy.032408.153621
52. Bullman TA, Kang HK. The risk of suicide among wounded Vietnam veterans. Am J Public Health. May 1996;86(5):662-667.
53. Braaten AJ, Parsons TD, McCue R, Sellers A, Burns WJ. Neurocognitive differential diagnosis of dementing diseases: Alzheimer's dementia, vascular dementia, frontotemporal dementia, and major depressive disorder. *Int J Neurosci.* 2006;116(11):1271-1293.
54. Coutinho AE, Chapman KE. The anti-inflammatory and immunosuppressive effects of glucocorticoids, recent developments and mechanistic insights. *Mol Cell Endocrinol.* Mar 15 2011;335(1):2-13. doi: 10.1016/j.mce.2010.04.005
55. Chen H, Lombès M, Le Menuet D. Glucocorticoid receptor represses brain-derived neurotrophic factor expression in neuron-like cells. *Mol Brain.* 2017;10(1):1-16.
56. Steffens DC, McQuoid DR, Payne ME, Potter GG. Change in hippocampal volume on magnetic resonance imaging and

cognitive decline among older depressed and nondepressed subjects in the neurocognitive outcomes of depression in the elderly study. *Am J Geriatr Psychiatry.* 2011;19(1):4-12.

57. Insulin Resistance and Diabetes. Centers for Disease Control and Prevention. Updated June 20, 2022. Accessed November 23, 2022. https://www.cdc.gov/diabetes/basics/insulin-resistance
58. What is Diabetes? Centers for Disease Control and Prevention. Updated December 16, 2021. https://www.cdc.gov/diabetes/basics/diabetes.html
59. Goldstein BJ. Insulin resistance as the core defect in type 2 diabetes mellitus. *Am J Card.* 2002;90(5):3-10.
60. Menezes Zanoveli J, de Morais H, Caroline da Silva Dias I, Karoline Schreiber A, Pasquini de Souza C, Maria da Cunha J. Depression associated with diabetes: from pathophysiology to treatment. *Curr Diabetes Rev.* 2016;12(3):165-178.
61. Strachan MW, Reynolds RM, Marioni RE, Price JF. Cognitive function, dementia and type 2 diabetes mellitus in the elderly. *Nat Rev Endocrinol.* 2011;7(2):108-114.
62. Xu X, Mishra GD, Dobson AJ, Jones M. Progression of diabetes, heart disease, and stroke multimorbidity in middle-aged women: a 20-year cohort study. *PLoS Med.* 2018;15(3):e1002516.
63. Dregan A, Charlton J, Chowienczyk P, Gulliford MC. Chronic inflammatory disorders and risk of type 2 diabetes mellitus, coronary heart disease, and stroke: a population-based cohort study. *Circulation.* 2014;130(10):837-844.
64. Wu Y, He J, Sun X, et al. Carotid atherosclerosis and its relationship to coronary heart disease and stroke risk in patients with type 2 diabetes mellitus. *Medicine.* 2017;96(39).
65. Einarson TR, Acs A, Ludwig C, Panton UH. Prevalence of cardiovascular disease in type 2 diabetes: a systematic literature review of scientific evidence from across the world in 2007–2017. *Cardiovasc Diabetol.* 2018;17(1):1-19.
66. de Ritter R, de Jong M, Vos RC, et al. Sex differences in the risk of vascular disease associated with diabetes. *Biol Sex Differ.* 2020;11(1):1-11.
67. Whitmer RA, Gilsanz P, Quesenberry CP, Karter AJ, Lacy ME. Association of type 1 diabetes and hypoglycemic and

hyperglycemic events and risk of dementia. *Neurology.* 2021;97(3):e275-e283.

68. Lacy ME, Gilsanz P, Karter AJ, Quesenberry CP, Pletcher MJ, Whitmer RA. Long-term glycemic control and dementia risk in type 1 diabetes. *Diabetes Care.* 2018;41(11):2339-2345.
69. Cholerton B, Baker LD, Craft S. Insulin, cognition, and dementia. *Eur J Pharmacol.* 2013;719(1-3):170-179.
70. McMillan JM, Mele BS, Hogan DB, Leung AA. Impact of pharmacological treatment of diabetes mellitus on dementia risk: systematic review and meta-analysis. *BMJ Open Diabetes Res Care.* 2018;6(1):e000563.
71. Weiner S. Hearing loss in diabetes often remains undiscussed. Endocrine Today. January 6, 2021. Accessed March 18, 2022. https://www.healio.com/news/endocrinology/20210105/hearing-loss-in-diabetes-often-remains-undiscussed
72. Rooth MA. The prevalence and impact of vision and hearing loss in the elderly. *N C Med J.* 2017;78(2):118-120.
73. Feher-Prout T. Stress and coping in families with deaf children. *J Deaf Stud Deaf Educ.* 1996;1(3):155-166.
74. Mitchell RE, Karchmer MA. Chasing the mythical ten percent: parental hearing status of deaf and hard of hearing students in the United States. *SLS.* 2004 Winter;4(2):138-163. doi:10.1353/sls.2004.0005
75. Holt-Lunstad J. The potential public health relevance of social isolation and loneliness: prevalence, epidemiology, and risk factors. *Public Policy & Aging Report.* 2017;27(4):127-130.
76. Yanguas J, Pinazo-Henandis S, Tarazona-Santabalbina FJ. The complexity of loneliness. *Acta Biomed.* 2018;89(2):302.
77. Rokach A. Loneliness in pre and post-operative cancer patients: a mini review. *Emerging Science Journal.* 2019;3(1):53-57.
78. Rico-Uribe LA, Caballero FF, Martín-María N, Cabello M, Ayuso-Mateos JL, Miret M. Association of loneliness with all-cause mortality: a meta-analysis. *PLoS One.* 2018;13(1):e0190033.
79. McClintock MK, Conzen SD, Gehlert S, Masi C, Olopade F. Mammary cancer and social interactions: identifying multiple environments that regulate gene expression throughout the

lifespan. *J Gerontol B: Psychol Sci Soc Sci.* 2005;60(Special_Issue_1):32-41.
80. Rosedale M. Survivor loneliness of women following breast cancer. *Oncol Nurs Forum.* 2009 Mar;36(2):175-83. doi:10.1188/09.ONF.175-183
81. Momtaz YA, Hamid TA, Yusoff S, et al. Loneliness as a risk factor for hypertension in later life. *J Aging Health.* 2012;24(4):696-710.
82. Petitte T, Mallow J, Barnes E, Petrone A, Barr T, Theeke L. A systematic review of loneliness and common chronic physical conditions in adults. *Open Psychol J.* 2015;8(Suppl 2):113.
83. Van Den Heuvel C, Thornton E, Vink R. Traumatic brain injury and Alzheimer's disease: a review. *Prog Brain Res.* 2007;161:303-316.
84. Cholerton B, Larson E, Baker LD, et al. Neuropathologic correlates of cognition in a population-based sample. *J Alzheimers Dis.* 2013;36(4):699-709.
85. Latimer CS, Keene CD, Flanagan ME, et al. Resistance to Alzheimer disease neuropathologic changes and apparent cognitive resilience in the Nun and Honolulu-Asia Aging Studies. *J Neuropathol Exp Neurol.* 2017;76(6):458-466.
86. Franzmeier N, Düzel E, Jessen F, et al. Left frontal hub connectivity delays cognitive impairment in autosomal-dominant and sporadic Alzheimer's disease. *Brain.* 2018;141(4):1186-1200.
87. Humphries T, Kushalnagar P, Mathur G, et al. Avoiding linguistic neglect of deaf children. *Soc Serv Rev.* 2016;90(4):589-619.
88. Skotara N, Salden U, Kügow M, Hänel-Faulhaber B, Röder B. The influence of language deprivation in early childhood on L2 processing: an ERP comparison of deaf native signers and deaf signers with a delayed language acquisition. *BMC Neurosci.* 2012;13(1):44-44. doi: 10.1186/1471-2202-13-44.
89. Mayberry RI, Davenport T, Roth A, Halgren E. Neurolinguistic processing when the brain matures without language. *Cortex.* 2018 Feb;99:390-403.

90. Anjum I, Fayyaz M, Wajid A, Sohail W, Ali A. Does obesity increase the risk of dementia: a literature review. *Cureus.* 2018;10(5).
91. Sahathevan R. Dementia: An overview of risk factors. In: Martin CR, Preedy VR, eds. *Diet and Nutrition in Dementia and Cognitive Decline.* Elsevier;2015:187-198.
92. Günak MM, Billings J, Carratu E, Marchant NL, Favarato G, Orgeta V. Post-traumatic stress disorder as a risk factor for dementia: systematic review and meta-analysis. *Br J Psychiatry.* 2020;217(5):600-608. doi: 10.1192/bjp.2020.150

PART III:
THE HEARING LOSS AND DEMENTIA CONNECTION

In a 2013 study published by John Hopkins University, researchers followed over 2,000 elderly adults for 6 years. At the end of the study, participants with severe hearing loss were 24% more likely to see cognitive decline than their peers without hearing loss. Other studies have found that the more significant an individual's hearing loss is, the higher the likelihood of cognitive decline. There are several explanations for the hearing loss and dementia connection. For the details, read on.

CHAPTER 4
HEARING LOSS AS A RISK FACTOR FOR DEMENTIA

"Not to brag or anything, but I can forget what I am doing while I am doing it."

Author Unknown

Let's get right to the heart of the mystery regarding the hearing loss and dementia connection. Why in the world would hearing loss be associated with dementia? The answer is somewhat complex but can be viewed through a simple metaphorical framework.

The simple explanation relates to the concept of cognitive reserve. Cognitive reserve refers to the brain's ability to adapt to aging changes over time.[1] Some individuals, including myself, have a hearing loss due to a specific etiology (cause) or combination of etiological factors. Common etiologies for hearing loss include rubella, cytomegalovirus (CMV), or meningitis.[2,3] Various etiologies—including unknown causes of hearing loss—can sometimes lead to a lower cognitive reserve than someone who might otherwise not have a condition that results in sensory loss.

To help with understanding cognitive reserve, let's consider an illustrative example. If we have a fancy sports car with six gears, we could compare this to a pickup truck, which generally has fewer gears (commonly four gears). The sports car's six gears allow it to go much faster than the pickup truck with fewer gears. When the need for acceleration arises, the sports car is more likely to meet the challenge because it has more gears or options to employ. The pickup truck, even when functioning at its best, runs out of options first, maxing out at four gears. The starting design at the factory has a big impact on the vehicle's final abilities on the road. An individual without a primary organic etiology resulting in a "vulnerability factor" is higher on the ladder rung of cognitive reserve. In terms of dementia risk, these individuals with fewer to no vulnerability factors have much more room to fall in terms of dementia onset. This is as opposed to an organic vulnerability that lends itself a shorter distance to the threshold of dementia.

It is as if an individual with hearing loss has less cash in the bank to make a down payment on a home. The less money for a down payment, the less home one can afford. The individual without any prior organic etiological factors affecting the cerebral cortex could have "more funds" for a down payment on a home and, thus, qualify for a bigger house. The smaller the home, the less room for error or manifestations of cognitive decline. The bigger the home, the more room for error before the cognitive decline is noted.

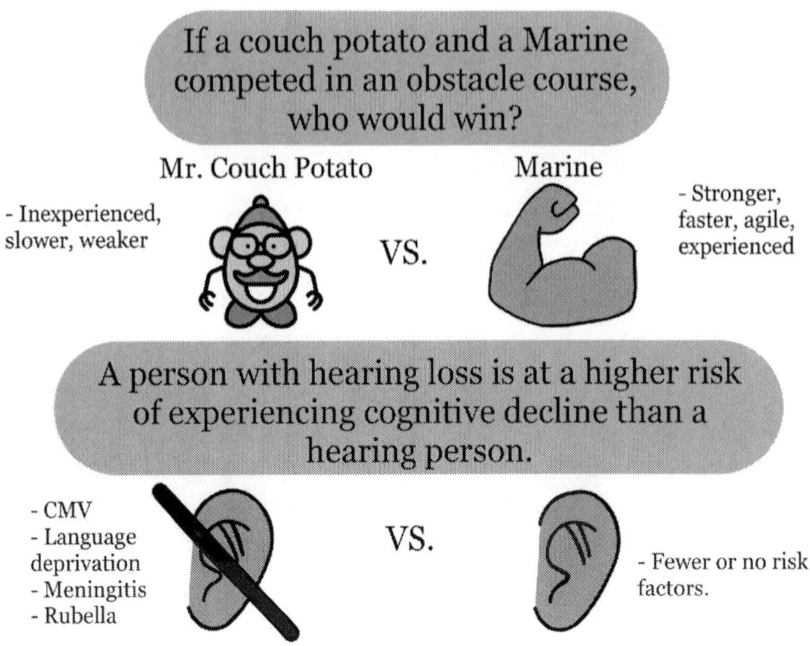

Another way of looking at this is to consider a hypothetical spur-of-the-moment obstacle course race between a U.S. Marine and someone we'll call "Mr. Couch Potato." Who is going to win the race? If you said, "Marine," I'd have to agree. Although Mr. Couch Potato and the Marine might have the same heart and motivation to win the obstacle course race, the Marine clearly has a head start in his physical training and has built up the stamina to endure and efficiently win the race. The Marine might go dancing at the local club afterward, while Mr. Couch Potato might likely go home and flop right back on the couch. The Marine represents those with a higher cognitive (or physical) reserve in contrast to Mr. Couch Potato.

Another common hearing loss etiology relates to newborns in the neonatal intensive care unit (NICU) who receive antibiotic therapy. Antibiotics of the aminoglycosides class are known to be associated with ototoxicity.[4] Ototoxicity is the development of hearing or balance problems due to a medication. Common aminoglycoside antibiotics include neomycin, amikacin (Amikin), gentamicin (Garamycin), streptomycin, and tobramycin (Tobi).

Administration of aminoglycosides is more common than you might think. One statistic shows that 80% of babies admitted to the NICU receive aminoglycosides. My wife is one example; she has a severe hearing loss with an etiology ascribed to gentamicin administration. It is estimated that adults given aminoglycosides may experience some degree of hearing loss ranging from mild to profound with a prevalence rate between 20-60%.[5]

Aside from hearing loss, research has shown that antibiotic treatments below age two are associated with an increased likelihood of a condition such as asthma, eczema, hay fever, food allergies, obesity, or ADHD.[6] The finding of an association of antibiotic treatments with a condition was analyzed from data involving over 14,500 children, with 70% of these children having received at least one antibiotic.

Do the ototoxic effects of antibiotics mean we avoid these medications like the plague? Not necessarily. The use of antibiotics must be weighed carefully with the pros and cons of a given condition being treated. Antibiotics and antiviral medications can be a boon for conditions that may be life-threatening and for which no other treatment exists.

Unfortunately, the cognitive reserve explanation for the hearing loss-dementia connection is not the be-all, end-all etiological factor. The hearing loss-dementia connection is further complicated by the fact that there are different types of hearing loss (eg, late onset vs. early onset) and communication modality preferences (vocal-auditory vs. American Sign Language).

For example, consider individuals who grow up identifying with Deaf culture, using ASL or other signed languages as their primary means of communication. Where do these individuals fit in terms of potential etiological factors associated with cognitive decline? Simply put, those individuals who experience dementia onset might fit into one of three etiological categories:

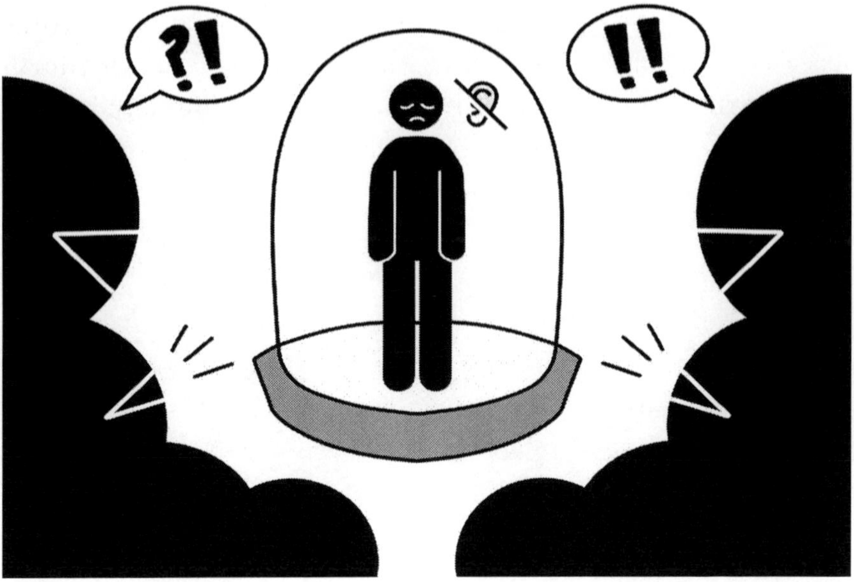

1. Cognitive reserve limitations brought on by one of the issues previously described (ie, meningitis, organic birth injury).
2. Language deprivation.
3. Other (eg, increased genetic susceptibility, substance misuse, social isolation).

While we have discussed cognitive reserve and its association with vulnerability factors, we haven't touched on language deprivation. As its name suggests, language deprivation refers to individuals with hearing loss who are deprived of exposure to a reliable language until well past the age window of optimal language acquisition. Also known as the critical period, the window for maximum language acquisition is in the first few years of life between birth to 5 years of age.[7,8]

Associated with language deprivation is something the academic literature describes as information deprivation, in which a deaf individual may have early exposure to a reliable language (ie, a visual language, such as sign language) but lack full access to incidental learning opportunities.[9] This lack of information access is also associated with trauma related to unpredictability and a sense of loss of control in one's life.

As an example, Schild and Dalenberg found in their study that for many deaf individuals, their first earthquake experience—which in most cases was a minor incident without any injuries or destruction—was one of their three worst life experiences. Often referenced to as information deprivation trauma, the lack of information or knowledge of this naturally occurring event was believed to make it less predictable and less controllable.[9,10]

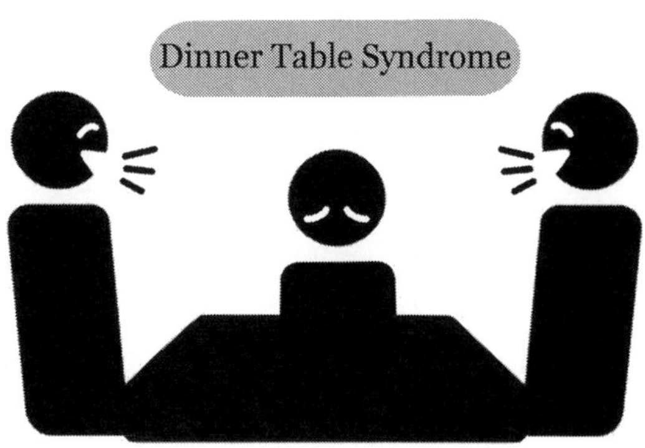

Moreover, many deaf individuals cannot access information from audio sources such as a radio to learn more about the extent of a disaster or possibly the well-being of family members. Dinner Table Syndrome—in which deaf members are excluded from family conversations due to difficulties deciphering the rapid communication that can occur among hearing individuals—is another example of limited incidental learning that can result in information deprivation.[11,12]

When we consider that most deaf children are born to hearing parents, the risk of language deprivation for this subgroup of individuals begins to make sense. Well-meaning hearing parents may receive and implement generally misguided information from the medical system's pathological model.[13] The medical system's pathological model centers on "fixing" hearing loss through hearing assistive devices, such as hearing aids and cochlear implants.

The pathological model may also emphasize the use of only vocal-auditory approaches to communication. Again, well-intentioned parents may pursue speech therapy services to maximize vocal-auditory skills. The pathological model needs to consider the fact that vocal-auditory methods are largely inaccessible to the majority of individuals with hearing loss. The lack of access to reliable visual language results in missing the critical period of language development.

Not only does language deprivation lead to alienation at home, it can also lead to disconnection from essentially all communities. This includes the culturally Deaf community, which can result in unnecessary social isolation that we know is a risk factor for cognitive decline. Indeed, one of the strengths of the deaf community is its vibrant and robust connections through social, political, sports, and other formal organizations. To experience language deprivation is to be cut off from what amounts to a critical protective factor, that of the deaf community.

Aside from the cognitive reserve explanation for the hearing loss-dementia connection, three other potential factors have been

> The lack of stimulation to a given area of the brain—in this case, the temporal lobe (with its associated memory functions)—can result in atrophy of that area. The muscles of the human body follow the same principle!

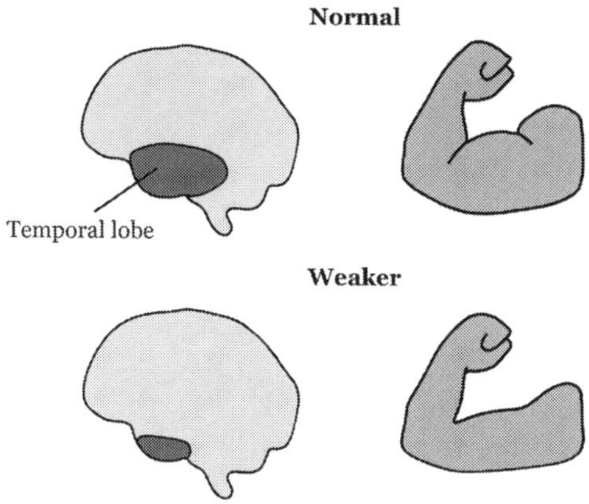

floated in the research. We'll quickly review these three etiological factors and then summarize the research findings that substantiate the hearing loss-dementia connection.

Three Other Potential Etiological Factors

The three other potential etiological factors for the hearing loss-dementia connection include structural changes to the brain, cognitive overload, and social isolation.

Structural Changes to the Brain. Longitudinal MRI studies have shown hearing loss to be associated with increased rates of brain volume loss. The brain volume loss seems to focus on the temporal lobe area, which includes the hippocampus—or, as we may recall, the brain's memory center. These findings suggest that hearing loss may also be associated with increased brain aging and nervous system decline.[14]

It needs to be clarified the exact mechanism by which hearing loss may be associated with increased rates of brain volume loss. The cascade hypothesis seems to be most applicable to individuals with mid-life or late-onset hearing loss. The essence

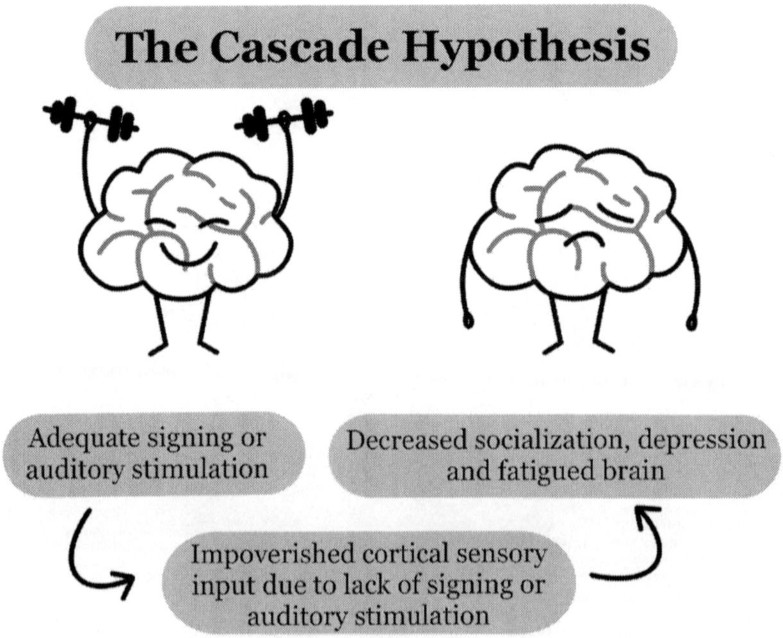

of the cascade hypothesis is that the areas of the brain that were stimulated before hearing loss onset begin to "waste away" due to the lack of ongoing stimulation.[15,16]

The cascade hypothesis is grounded in sensory deprivation. Just like muscles can weaken from lack of exercise, the unused parts of the brain become more fragile, which may lead to poorer memory functioning and, thus, dementia symptoms.

We must also consider some of the research which suggests that hearing loss may be associated with a particular type of dementia. As we have discussed, the four most common dementia types are Alzheimer's, vascular, Lewy body, and frontotemporal dementia. Some evidence suggests that Lewy body dementia may be the most common type associated with hearing loss.[15] However, repetition of these early studies needs to be conducted before any full-drawn conclusion can be made.

Cognitive Overload. Simply stated, the cognitive overload theory is the idea of the brain being "too busy" trying to comprehend communication that it neglects the other memory or thinking

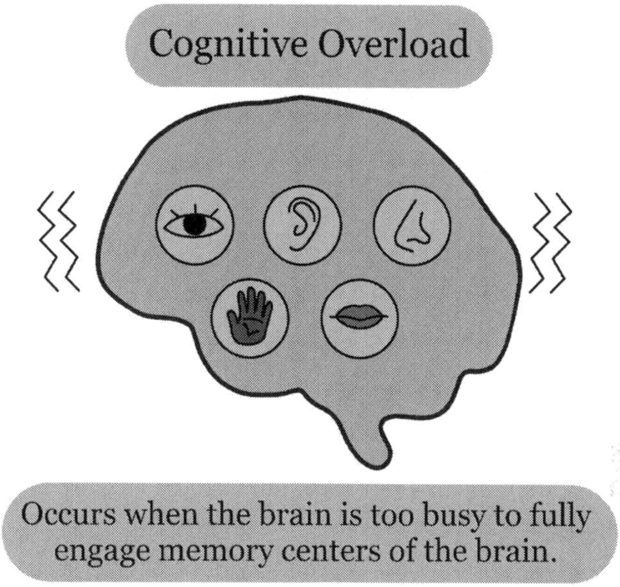

parts of its structures. Neglecting the memory and thinking parts of the brain can result in sensory deprivation, causing these unused areas to decline or weaken.

An additional framework for the cognitive overload theory is in the context of an individual's hearing loss type and life experiences. For example, for the individual with midlife or late-onset hearing loss, auditory signals sent to the brain may be fragmented or weak. These auditory signals may not be comprehended within the same auditory circuits before hearing loss onset. Instead, the brain may recruit other areas and divert more energy to decode or make sense of this poorer auditory signal. This extra load on the brain may limit how well the brain can buffer against other pathologic changes that can bring on dementia conditions.[17]

On the other hand, brain neuroimaging studies reflect less cognitive activity in specific language-related brain anatomical areas for those with congenital or early onset hearing loss who experience language deprivation during the formative developmental years. These neuroimaging studies show fewer "active hot spots" during communication.[18] In addition to less cognitive activity, aberrant brain areas are activated in those with language deprivation compared to those without language deprivation.[19]

With fewer available cognitive resources to assist with effective communication, the language-deprived brain has a lower level of cognitive reserve. Additionally, the language-deprived brain has limited cognitive resources to effectively "recruit and aid" with communication dynamics. The limited cognitive resources may come at the expense of other areas of cognition (eg, working memory) and contribute to mental health difficulties.[20] The constant overload of brain recruitment may again limit the brain's protective factors, increasing the risk of neurodegenerative disease onset.

Social Isolation. Social isolation is an excellent example of how hearing loss may not cause dementia but may contribute to an increased risk of dementia onset. As we learned in the previous chapter, social isolation has long been recognized as a strong predictor of dementia.[21-23]

Studies have demonstrated that hearing loss can lead to increased social isolation.[24] Compared to those who did not report hearing loss, the odds of experiencing psychological distress increased with the degree of hearing loss. There were 47% higher odds of depression due to the long-term repercussions brought on by the psychological distress of hearing loss.[25]

Communication barriers brought on by hearing loss can deter individuals from engaging in socialization opportunities or previously enjoyed activities. After all, with the mental and physical exhaustion that can come from straining to make sense of what others are saying, it's not surprising that many choose to forgo social activities and stay home.

Research Findings Associated with the Hearing Loss-Dementia Connection

Since the 1980s, multiple studies with large data sets and rigorous epidemiologic methodology have shown strong associations between hearing loss and dementia.[26,27] It is important to emphasize that there is a difference between hearing loss being a cause of dementia and hearing loss increasing the risk for dementia. Although prior research shows a strong association between hearing loss and dementia, it does not mean that hearing loss causes dementia. Instead, it would be more appropriate to say that hearing loss may contribute to the increased risk of dementia.

With each new study and each passing year, we have consistent findings of hearing loss being associated with increased dementia risk. One could say that we have come quite a way since the 1980s—nearly half a century. The literature has also exploded in recent years, giving us increased confidence to say that hearing loss does increase the risk for dementia.

A study that showed the association of cognitive decline with hearing loss was conducted by Dr. Frank Lin and his colleagues.[28] Dr. Lin looked at cognitive decline among 1,984 adults with an average age of 77. Cognitive measures were performed in years 1, 5, 8, 10, and 11. The combined outcome measures showed that adults with hearing loss had an average of 37% annual rate of cognitive decline when compared to those with normal hearing.

Additionally, Dr. Lin found that as hearing loss increased, the risk of dementia increased. Incident dementia increased across mild, moderate, and severe hearing loss levels. Mild hearing loss is thought to be associated with a doubled risk for dementia, with severe hearing loss leading to five times the risk for dementia.[29]

Other well-designed studies with large numbers of participants have confirmed the findings of Lin and his colleagues.[30-34] These studies were also conducted over multiple years. For instance, Dr. Jennifer Deal and her colleagues studied 2,304 adults over nine years. That study found that those with moderate hearing loss were noted to have an increased risk of dementia compared to those without hearing loss. Another study confirmed the prior findings over a more extended period of 17 years.[35] Hearing loss was also found by the Lancet Commission to be the most significant modifiable risk factor for dementia.[27]

Are There Other Explanations for the Hearing Loss and Dementia Connection?

One criticism raised in the literature is whether there might be a sort of "reverse causality" taking place; rather than hearing loss increasing the risk for dementia, the cognitive decline might be contributing to false positive findings of peripheral hearing loss.[36] For instance, consider the idea that hearing tests can be cognitively demanding, especially for an individual with cognitive decline. Could the inability to engage in audiology testing procedures lead to an artificially deflated audiogram rather than true hearing loss? Although a reasonable hypothesis, it doesn't stand up to the consistent and repeated findings from the multiple longitudinal studies that indicate hearing loss onset before any known cognitive decline.

Another essential factor is how cognitive decline is measured in individuals with hearing loss. Two crucial considerations in this area of research are: 1) using a cognitive task that does not rely on auditory input to complete the task; and 2) ensuring the use of objective measures as opposed to self-report measures of cognitive decline. The latter's importance is essential due to the general tendency of individuals with dementia to lack awareness of their own memory difficulties.[37] The very, very few studies that have refuted the hearing loss and dementia connection are poorly designed studies that essentially fail to follow at least one or both of the above essential considerations in studying the hearing loss and dementia connection.

Do Hearing Assistive Devices Help Prevent or Delay Dementia Onset?

You might wonder whether hearing aids or cochlear implants would help lessen the risk of dementia onset. Isn't it nice to consider something—anything—that might delay or decrease the risk of dementia onset? We do not yet have enough research data that supports the idea of hearing aids or cochlear implants being the direct causal link for lessening the risk of dementia onset.[38,39] What do we mean by this?

Although hearing aids or cochlear implants may stimulate the brain and potentially help reduce social isolation, we also have to remember that variables associated with hearing aid or cochlear implant ownership can also be a protective factor. For example, those with hearing aids or cochlear implants may belong to a higher socioeconomic class. Those within a higher socioeconomic class may be at lower risk of cognitive decline and dementia.[40,41] Such a confounding variable can make it difficult to draw conclusions ascribed solely to the sensory rehabilitation treatment or mental stimulus thought to be provided by hearing aid and cochlear implant usage.[39]

With that said, it is interesting to note that at least one research article by Mamo et al. found that individuals with late-onset hearing loss with severe depression showed improvement in their symptoms one-month post implementation of a hearing assistive device.[42] The same authors of this study further suggested that the use of hearing assistive devices can be an attractive option in that it represents a low-risk, non-pharmacological intervention with at least some potential for reward.

If we are to use hearing assistive devices as a potential means of improving our social connections with others, it is important to track our hearing ability by engaging in at least annual audiology testing. Like tracking other healthcare metrics, such as blood pressure, cholesterol, and weight, hearing loss levels can be an important metric to follow to optimize our health. Moreover, data indicate that most individuals with late-onset hearing loss who could benefit from a hearing assistive device do not use them. Only 30% of hard of hearing adults ages 70+ reported using a hearing assistive device, with only 16% of a younger subset of adults indicating use of an assistive device.[43]

The potential for reward centers on the enhancement of social connections through the prospective improvement—and restoration—of communication comprehension that hearing assistive devices might bring. It is essential, however, to remember that improving social connections does not always come in the form of hearing assistive devices. As we have been discussing throughout this book, there is a large community of individuals who identify as Deaf and use a shared visual language (ASL) for communication. As a language minority, this community has a keen sense of shared place. This is part of the reason that hearing accommodations that might be touted as "quick fixes" for individuals with hearing loss do not apply in all cases. The deaf community is the social connection that someone with late-onset hearing loss may miss.

The Bottom Line

Effectively adapting to circumstances as an individual with hearing loss plays a crucial role in healthy aging. In essence, this includes learning how to interact effectively with others regardless of the limitations that hearing loss can bring. Yes, it can be a tall order for some of us. But it is a difficult task that must be conquered, and there are many creative ways to climb the seemingly insurmountable wall.

Learning to interact effectively with hearing loss does not just include the obvious, such as using hearing aids, or cochlear implants. For example, multiple automated speech recognition (ASR) software apps are available. These apps can be downloaded on one's smartphone, and conveniently used as needed. There are also ASR apps that will continue to work, albeit not as accurately, even when there is no Internet or cellular reception.

Adapting to circumstances as an individual with hearing loss requires stepping outside of one's comfort zone as you persist in trying your best to engage with others. Let's also remember the importance of immersing oneself in stimulating hobbies for the mind and body. The importance of adaptation applies to all levels of hearing loss, including those who communicate using ASL as their primary communication medium.

Let's go into further detail regarding how we can best adapt to circumstances as an individual with hearing loss. Our ability to adapt to circumstances can, in the long run, translate into a means of delaying dementia onset. We turn to these "brain protectants" in the next chapter.

Key Takeaways

The statistics for individuals with hearing loss are staggering, especially among older adults. The latest numbers indicate that approximately half of all adults over 60 have a hearing loss of at least 25 dB. These numbers amount to around 38 million Americans. And with the aging demographics, this number is likely to double to 74 million by 2060.[14,43]

Along with a more significant proportion of our population experiencing hearing loss, there is an alarming rise in the prevalence of dementia worldwide. Estimates indicate that at least 32% of the population will experience dementia. These findings become even more intriguing when we consider that those with hearing loss are estimated to experience an 18% to 40% accelerated risk of cognitive decline.[28,44] Disappointing, huh?

Various theories discussed in this chapter lend themselves to the increased risk of hearing loss-associated cognitive decline. These theories include reduced cognitive reserve brought on by the condition causing the hearing loss, structural changes to the brain due to decreased stimulation of the auditory cortex, and increased cognitive load brought on by the energy needed to decode speech.

The importance of recognizing hearing loss as a risk factor as opposed to being a causal factor was emphasized. For example, social withdrawal brought on by one's hearing loss can trigger a cascade of social isolation, psychological distress, and myriad health issues that can lead to cognitive decline.

In the next chapter, we discuss things we can do to reduce the dementia risk factor, including adapting to circumstances as an individual with hearing loss. Let's cash in on those "brain-protective" factors.

CHAPTER FOUR REFERENCES

1. Stern Y. What is cognitive reserve? Theory and research application of the reserve concept. *J Int Neuropsychol Soc.* 2002;8(3):448-460.
2. Roizen NJ. Etiology of hearing loss in children: nongenetic causes. *Pediatr Clin North Am.* 1999;46(1):49-64.
3. Morzaria S, Westerberg BD, Kozak FK. Systematic review of the etiology of bilateral sensorineural hearing loss in children. *Int J Pediatr Otorhinolaryngol.* 2004;68(9):1193-1198
4. O'neil WG. Aminoglycoside induced ototoxicity. *Toxicology.* 2008;249(2-3):91-96.
5. Szczepek AJ. Ototoxicity:old and new foes. In: Hatzopoulos S, ed. *Advances in Clinical Audiology.* InTech; 2017. https://www.intechopen.com/chapters/53540
6. Aversa Z, Atkinson EJ, Schafer MJ, et al. Association of infant antibiotic exposure with childhood health outcomes. *Mayo Clin Proc.* 2021;96(1):66-77. doi: 10.1016/j.mayocp.2020.07.019.
7. Mayberry RI. The critical period for language acquisition and the deaf child's language comprehension: a psycholinguistic approach. *Bulletin d'Audiophonologie.* 1998;14:349-360.
8. Speech and language developmental milestones. National Institute on Deafness and Other Communication Disorders. Updated October 13, 2022. Accessed December 12, 2022. https://www.nidcd.nih.gov/health/speech-and-language
9. Schild S, Dalenberg CJ. Trauma exposure and traumatic symptoms in deaf adults. *Psychol Trauma.* 2012;4(1):117.
10. Carlson EB, Dalenberg CJ. A conceptual framework for the impact of traumatic experiences. *Trauma Viol Abuse.* 2000;1(1):4-28.
11. Hall WC, Smith SR, Sutter EJ, DeWindt LA, Dye TD. Considering parental hearing status as a social determinant of deaf population health: insights from experiences of the "dinner table syndrome." *PLoS One.* 2018;13(9):e0202169.
12. Meek DR. Dinner table syndrome: A phenomenological study of deaf individuals' experiences with inaccessible communication. *The Qualitative Report.* 2020;25(6):1676A-1694.

13. Wilson JA, Atcherson SR. Audism and its implications for audiology. *Perspectives of the ASHA Special Interest Groups.* 2017;2(8).
14. Mueller G. 20Q: Hearing Loss and Dementia-Highlights from Key Research. 2019.
15. Jung J, Bae SH, Han JH, et al. Relationship between hearing loss and dementia differs according to the underlying mechanism. *J Clin Neurol.* 2021;17(2):290. doi: 10.3988/jcn.2021.17.2.290.
16. Uchida Y, Sugiura S, Nishita Y, Saji N, Sone M, Ueda H. Age-related hearing loss and cognitive decline—The potential mechanisms linking the two. *Auris Nasus Larynx.* 2019;46(1):1-9.
17. Griffiths TD, Lad M, Kumar S, et al. How can hearing loss cause dementia? *Neuron.* 2020 Nov 11;108(3):401-412. doi: 10.1016/j.neuron.2020.08.003
18. Gulati S. Language deprivation syndrome. In: Glickman NS, Hall WC, eds. *Language Deprivation and Deaf Mental Health.* Routledge; 2018:24-53.
19. Cheng Q, Roth A, Halgren E, Mayberry RI. Effects of early language deprivation on brain connectivity: language pathways in deaf native and late first-language learners of American Sign Language. *Front Hum Neurosci.* 2019;13:320.
20. Hall WC, Levin LL, Anderson ML. Language deprivation syndrome: a possible neurodevelopmental disorder with sociocultural origins. *Soc Psychiatry Psychiatr Epidemiol.* 2017;52(6):761-776.
21. Rutherford BR, Brewster K, Golub JS, Kim AH, Roose SP. Sensation and psychiatry: linking age-related hearing loss to late-life depression and cognitive decline. *Am J Psychiatry.* 2018;175(3):215-224.
22. Maharani A, Pendleton N, Leroi I. Hearing impairment, loneliness, social isolation, and cognitive function: longitudinal analysis using English longitudinal study on aging. *Am J Geriatr Psychiatry.* 2019;27(12):1348-1356.
23. Rafnsson SB, Orrell M, d'Orsi E, Hogervorst E, Steptoe A. Loneliness, social integration, and incident dementia over 6 years: prospective findings from the English Longitudinal Study of Ageing. *J Gerontology B.* 2020;75(1):114-124.

24. Suen J, Shukla A, Goman A, Price C, Lin F, Reed N. Associations between hearing loss, loneliness, and social isolation: a systematic review. *Innovation in Aging.* 2020;4:318-318. doi:10.1093/geroni/igaa057.1018
25. Abrams HB. Hearing loss and comorbidities: 2022 update. Adult Hearing. Accessed October 12, 2022. https://adulthearing.com/wp-content/uploads/2022/05/Hearing-Loss-and-Comorbidities-2022-Update.pdf
26. Uhlmann RF, Larson EB, Rees TS, Koepsell TD, Duckert LG. Relationship of hearing impairment to dementia and cognitive dysfunction in older adults. *JAMA.* 1989 Apr 7;261(13):1916-1919.
27. Livingston G, Huntley J, Sommerlad A, et al. Dementia prevention, intervention, and care: 2020 report of the Lancet Commission. *Lancet.* 2020;396(10248):413-446. doi: 10.1016/s0140-6736(20)30367-6
28. Lin FR, Yaffe K, Xia J, et al. Hearing loss and cognitive decline in older adults. *JAMA Intern Med.* 2013;173(4):293-299.
29. The link between hearing loss and Alzheimer's. Lucid Hearing blog. Accessed October 19, 2022. https://shop.lucidhearing.com/how-supporting-your-hearing-supports-your-memory-too-the-link-between-hearing-loss-and-alzheimers/
30. Loughrey DG, Kelly ME, Kelley GA, Brennan S, Lawlor BA. Association of age-related hearing loss with cognitive function, cognitive impairment, and dementia: a systematic review and meta-analysis. *JAMA Otolaryngol Head Neck Surg.* 2018;144(2):115-126.
31. Loughrey DG, Feeney J, Kee F, et al. Social factors may mediate the relationship between subjective age-related hearing loss and episodic memory. *Aging Ment Health.* 2021;25(5):824-831.
32. Deal JA, Betz J, Yaffe K, et al. Hearing impairment and incident dementia and cognitive decline in older adults: the health ABC study. *J Gerontol A Biomed Sci Med Sci.* 2017;72(5):703-709.
33. Thomson RS, Auduong P, Miller AT, Gurgel RK. Hearing loss as a risk factor for dementia: a systematic review. *Laryngoscope Investig Otolaryngol.* 2017;2(2):69-79.

34. Gurgel RK, Ward PD, Schwartz S, Norton MC, Foster NL, Tschanz JT. Relationship of hearing loss and dementia: a prospective, population-based study. *Otol Neurotol.* 2014;35(5):775.
35. Gallacher J, Ilubaera V, Ben-Shlomo Y, et al. Auditory threshold, phonologic demand, and incident dementia. *Neurology.* 2012;79(15):1583-1590.
36. Wayne RV, Johnsrude IS. A review of causal mechanisms underlying the link between age-related hearing loss and cognitive decline. *Ageing Res Rev.* 2015;23:154-166.
37. Wilcox JA, Duffy PR. Is it a senior moment or early dementia? Addressing memory concerns in older patients. *Curr Psychiatry.* 2016;15(5):28-35.
38. Dawes P, Tye-Murray N, McCreery R, Alexander JM, Chermak G, McCaslin DL. 20Q: Hearing loss and dementia—Association, link or causation? *Audiology Online.* 2017.
39. Mahmoudi E, Basu T, Langa K, et al. Can hearing aids delay time to diagnosis of dementia, depression, or falls in older adults? *J Am Geriatr Soc.* 2019;67(11):2362-2369.
40. Goldbourt U, Schnaider-Beeri M, Davidson M. Socioeconomic status in relationship to death of vascular disease and late-life dementia. *J Neurol Sci.* 2007;257(1-2):177-181.
41. Deckers K, Cadar D, van Boxtel MP, Verhey FR, Steptoe A, Köhler S. Modifiable risk factors explain socioeconomic inequalities in dementia risk: evidence from a population-based prospective cohort study. *J Alzheimers Dis.* 2019;71(2):549-557.
42. Mamo SK, Reed NS, Price C, et al. Hearing loss treatment in older adults with cognitive impairment: a systematic review. *J Speech Lang Hear Res.* 2018;61(10):2589-2603.
43. Beck DL. Aging, hearing, cognition, and neuropsychology: interview with Boaz M. Ben-David, PhD. The Hearing Review. November 1, 2021. Accessed October 28, 2022. https://hearingreview.com/inside-hearing/people/hearing-15
44. Ford AH, Hankey GJ, Yeap BB, Golledge J, Flicker L, Almeida OP. Hearing loss and the risk of dementia in later life. *Maturitas.* 2018;112:1-11.

PART IV: **MITIGATING THE DEMENTIA RISK FACTORS**

In previous chapters, we discussed the risk factors for dementia. We will now discuss specific ways to protect that precious invaluable brain resting upon our necks. Because there continues to be no specific medical treatment for eradicating dementia, prevention strategies offer the best weapons against the disease.

Remember the story in the first chapter about my family's 2019 summer road trip? Before hiking to see the petroglyphs, the ranger briefed us on the trail's rules. She explained the importance of not touching the petroglyphs or stirring up dust near the historic sites. These rules help protect the ancient rock artwork. Much like we can protect these historical artifacts, we can also be proactive to form somewhat of a shield to protect our brains.

This chapter will explore specific tools you can use to keep your brain as healthy as possible. It is a healthy brain that is the best defense against dementia. Are you ready? Let's take the plunge!

CHAPTER FIVE
PROTECTING THE BRAIN

"Your mind needs exercise just as much as your body does . . . that's why I simply think of jogging every day."
Author Unknown

The first thing that you can do to help ward off dementia is one that brings dread and despair to many individuals. This dementia-warding-off factor has occasionally been referred to by only its first letter, or even worse, The "Scary E": exercise!

Brain Protectant #1: Exercise

For those who hate to exercise, I apologize for opening this chapter with the "Scary E" as one of the protective factors for healthy brain longevity. It is true, though, that exercise is one of the best and most crucial brain protectants.[1-3] Perhaps you are wondering... wouldn't it be nice if we could simply do as the quote for this chapter says (ie, merely think of jogging to reap the benefits of exercise)? I think we all wish it were that simple and easy. Unfortunately, reaping the actual benefits of exercise is maximized when it is intentional and consistent.[4]

Often referred to as a lifestyle modification means of reducing dementia risk, it's important to note that there are many creative ways to get your exercise in. Take heart, folks. Exercise does not have to be painful or tedious. Some creative means of exercising include walking the dog, doing water aerobics, or riding a bike.

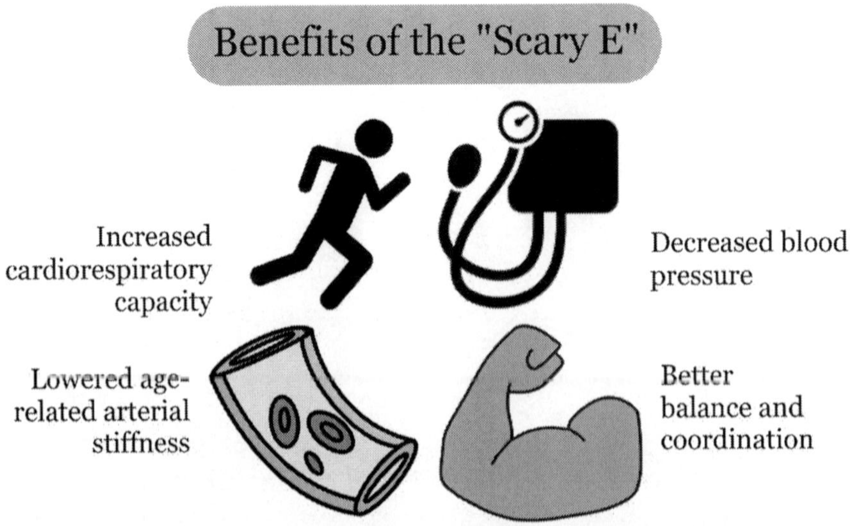

Although exercising to the point of breaking a sweat may benefit overall health, sweating is not always required. Something as simple as walking has also been found to do wonders for one's health. One study found that a daily walk could reduce the risk of dementia by a whopping 40%.[5] It's a fact of life—physical activity assists us with optimizing our cognitive functioning and general health in a way unparalleled to many medications or supplements.[6-9]

Perhaps you want to engage in an exercise routine but want to know if there is a "best of the best" out of the seemingly countless programs available. One study pooled together 39 other studies that involved various exercise types such as tai chi and resistance strength training to see if one modality stood above the rest.[10] All exercise modalities had positive effects, but the most robust evidence was for cross-training type programs that included an aerobics component. The finding of an aerobic element being an essential part of an exercise program for reserving cognitive function has also been confirmed by other studies.[11,12]

All things being equal, the program you pick should boil down to doing what you will most enjoy. And this is an important question to consider. Your enjoyment and satisfaction with your exercise routine determine your stick-to-it factor.[13,14] Another critical component is having a positive attitude with whatever you decide to do. In one study, participants having a positive attitude (eg, "exercise is fun") demonstrated higher adherence to their exercise routine (80%) than participants with a negative attitude (a measly 24%) toward the routine (eg, "exercise is boring").

So, what's the moral of the story? The next time you are doing push-ups or jogging that first of several miles and thinking to yourself, "I hate this," catch yourself and rephrase it as, "I love this!"

Here's the thing: if you persist long enough in pushing positive thoughts while allowing yourself to experience the moment, you will eventually lend credence to those positive thoughts and embrace those moments.[15] This is all part of the cognitive bias mindset that seems counterintuitive and paradoxical. The deal here is that you must utilize at least some level of belief (even if it is just a teeny bit) in positive thoughts. Yes, it is possible to "trick your brain to enjoy the things you hate." If exercise has all of the health benefits that science claims it has, what's the harm in exercising (yes, there's the E word again!) an iota of belief that pushes us to embrace the "Scary E"?!

Final Words on Exercise as a Brain Protectant. The idea of exercise helping our cognitive facilities makes intuitive sense. We can think of the cardiovascular and metabolic benefits. These benefits may assist with addressing such adverse health factors as obesity, heart disease, and hypertension.[9,16-20] One recent study of 28,916 participants reinforces the literature on exercise's benefits in reducing dementia risk. The HUNT study found that weekly moderate-to-vigorous physical activity (breaking into a sweat) was associated with reduced dementia risk over a 25-year follow-up period.[21]

While exercising five days a week for at least 30 minutes each time can have astounding benefits for the mind and body, even exercising one or two days a week still has significant results.[10] The more days of exercise, the better—though you don't want to overexert yourself. Pay attention to how your body feels. It is also essential to check with your primary care provider before beginning any exercise regimen.

Brain Protectant #2: Nutrition

Along with exercise, nutrition is a vital part of the lifestyle modification options for preventing or delaying dementia onset. Eating healthy can prevent plaque buildup in arteries. Plaque buildup in arteries decreases oxygen flow to essential areas of your body, especially your brain.[22] In essence, plaque buildup can increase the risk of vascular dementia onset.[23]

Excess glucose (blood sugar) can cause inflammation in the arteries.[24] This is part of the reason that diabetes is considered a risk factor for dementia. Diabetes is linked with higher-than-average blood glucose, plaque buildup in the arteries, and associated inflammation.[25] In essence, a healthy diet is associated with approximately 40% improvement in cognition. It is also associated with a 30% reduction in depression. And this is all after controlling for education, income, other health behaviors, and body weight.[26] Adopting a healthy, nutritious approach to eating has been noted to cause differences in the gut microbiome (bacteria that live in digestive tracts) in as little as two to three weeks![27]

So what is considered a healthy, nutritious approach? The Mediterranean dietary approach to eating is one of the most studied and well-known dietary patterns worldwide. Research has found that following a Mediterranean approach to eating can not only help ward off dementia onset but result in a multitude of health benefits. These benefits include reducing stroke risks, cardiovascular disease, diabetes, and all-cause mortality.[28] A Mediterranean diet entails foods such as berries, nuts, vegetables, beans, dark chocolate, and seafood with omega-3 fatty acids. Seafood high in omega-3 fatty acids includes salmon (Atlantic and Chinook salmon varieties are higher in omega-3 than Chum, Coho,

Pink, and Sockeye varieties), sardines, tuna (Bluefin is higher than the Albacore variety), halibut, and trout.

Some people worry about mercury or other pollutants that might be associated with some seafood. Others simply don't like seafood. There are creative ways to address these concerns. Small fish like anchovies and sardines are essentially free of environmental toxins. They are also a great source of omega-3.[29] Smoked salmon, shrimp, and canned seafood can also carry less of the "fish taste."

The fascinating thing about the Mediterranean approach to eating is that even small changes in nutrition intake can pay enormous dividends for overall health. One study had participants eat two seafood meals a week, an extra half-serving of fruit a day, an extra serving of vegetables a day, and an extra serving of legumes (also known as pulses, which include lentils, peas, beans, chickpeas, and the like).[30] By incorporating these simple nutrition changes, the study participants ate fewer meals of highly processed foods, such as fried, sugary fast foods, and simple carbohydrates. The results also showed they ate significantly fewer meals while lowering their food costs by more than $100 per month. Talk about a simple way to improve overall brain health and naturally temper the occasional cravings we get for unhealthy food. We can turn this into a simple mantra: "Seafood, greens, nuts and beans, and a little dark chocolate." What a great place to start.

Swapping oil and butter for extra virgin olive oil is another easy, simple change. Extra virgin olive oil has a far higher antioxidant count than other cooking oils. Contrary to what you may have heard or read, olive oil does not lose its health benefits or become unhealthy when heated.[31]

While on the subject of unhealthy food items, we must be careful about diet sodas and artificial sweeteners. These items have been linked to higher rates of depression. And if that wasn't bad enough, animal studies have shown associations with hippocampal damage (which, as we know, would worsen memory).[32]

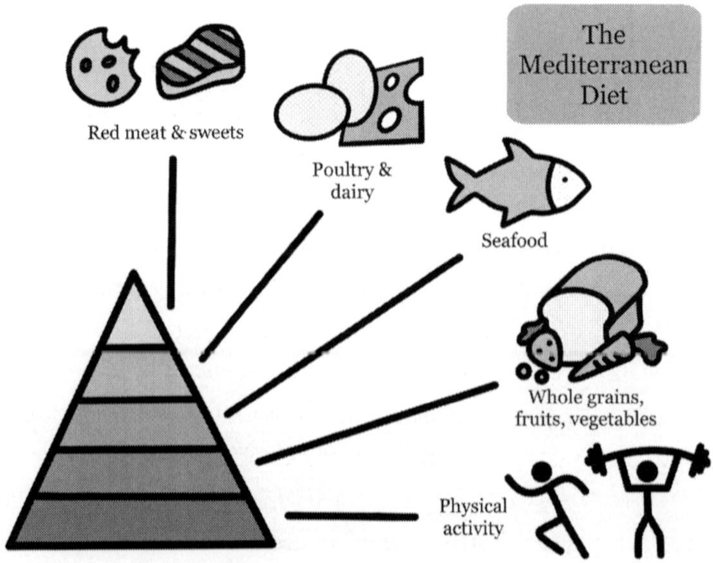

It may be surprising for some that dark chocolate is a staple at the healthy Mediterranean table. I recall fondly when my family and I had a long, hard laugh when my grandma defended her chocolate consumption habits. Grandma protested, "Chocolate is healthy for you!" Grandma was right—to an extent. It's not the high sugar in milk chocolate or white chocolate that is deemed to have the health benefits associated with the Mediterranean diet. It's dark chocolate. Dark chocolate, including cocoa, has a lot of polyphenols.[33] Polyphenols are antioxidants that have brain-protective effects. Antioxidants have polyphenols that can protect against weight gain through interactions with the gut microbiome. Polyphenols are also found in various berries. To this day, I happily take Grandma's sage advice as I seem to have inherited her profound love of chocolate.

Final Words on Nutrition as a Brain Protectant. Making small and simple changes in our nutrition intake weekly can add up over time and improve overall brain health. MyPlate Calorie Counter is one app that can help us make informed food choices. The app is available free from your smartphone's app store. The app can read barcodes on food packaging and give helpful nutrition information. Although the app's name sounds like it is strictly for counting calories, it is much more than that. Besides tracking nutrient intake, the app offers recipes, meal plans, and workout routines. A community section provides peer support, which can act as a source of motivation.

Simply put, Mediterranean foods are rich in nutrients long considered essential to brain functioning, such as magnesium, folate, and B-vitamins. Keep in mind that food sources provide benefits that simple supplements cannot. Crucial nutrients from food help increase brain-derived neurotrophic factors (BDNF), which improves neuroplasticity.[34] Recall also that the hippocampus is one of the brain structures that shrinks with age. As much as 60% of that atrophy may be related to the quality of one's diet.[35]

Inflammation is both a cause and consequence of cognitive decline and a host of mental health issues. Intentionally striving to engage in healthy eating habits can be a powerful weapon in fighting inflammation and maximizing and preserving cognitive function.

Brain Protectant #3: Blood Pressure Monitoring

Remember when we discussed high blood pressure (hypertension) as a risk factor for dementia? Multiple clinical research findings confirm that individuals with uncontrolled and untreated hypertension develop more white matter lesions than persons with controlled and treated hypertension.

Hypertension can lead to ischemia (low oxygen) or damage to myelinated neurons (white matter). The resulting white matter lesions are a strong predictor of cognitive decline. Higher frequencies of white matter lesions also increase the risk of stroke, dementia, and death in older adults.[36]

The use of antihypertensive agents not only lowers blood pressure but significantly reduces the risk of stroke and heart failure.[37,38] The risk of white matter disease is also reduced.[39]

Properly Taking Your Blood Pressure

30 minutes prior to taking your blood pressure reading, don't smoke, exercise, or drink caffeine or alcohol.

1. Relax in a chair and refrain from talking.
2. Use a properly calibrated and validated instrument; check the cuff size and fit.
3. Using your left arm on a flat surface at heart level, place the bottom of the blood pressure cuff above the end of the bend of the left elbow.
4. Record your results.

AM: Take **at least** two readings, 1 minute apart in the morning before medication.

PM: Repeat in the evening before dinner.

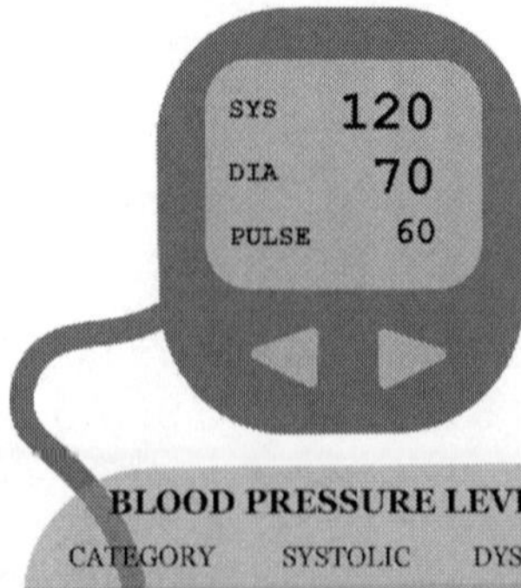

BLOOD PRESSURE LEVELS

CATEGORY	SYSTOLIC	DYSTOLIC
Normal	-120	-80
Elevated	120 - 129	-80
High - Stage 1	130 - 139	80-89
High - Stage 2	140+	90+
CRISIS	180+	120+

CONSULT YOUR DOCTOR IMMEDIATELY

Moreover, researchers have found that individuals who took three or more medications to aggressively lower hypertension were significantly less likely to develop dementia.[40]

It is crucial to be proactive in monitoring potential hypertension. One recommendation is to purchase a personal home blood pressure monitor. Digital blood pressure monitors are easy to use and can be purchased online or from most pharmacy stores. Today, these devices are reasonably affordable. You can check and track your blood pressure from home with a digital blood pressure monitor.

We are truly fortunate to live in a time with access to various digital blood pressure monitors with many features. Some devices can automatically send information over Wi-Fi to your doctor after each measurement. Sending your blood pressure statistics to your doctor can assist with medication management and treatment.

Monitoring blood pressure is essential because hypertension symptoms are not typically obvious or notable. Frequently referenced as a "silent killer," hypertension is usually not noted until organ damage is imminent or has already occurred.[41,42]

When should we be concerned with our blood pressure numbers? Blood pressure tends to be reported as a fraction. Generally speaking, if you have a top number (systolic blood pressure) falling between 130 and 180, you are strongly encouraged to go and get the medications you need to bring your blood pressure down below or as close as possible to 120.[43] Go get help—pronto!

The opposite of high blood pressure can also be problematic. Low blood pressure or hypotension (usually less than 120/75 mmHg) can worsen cognitive functioning.[44] In fact, cognitive decline itself has also been linked to hypotension. Hypotension can result from overly aggressive treatment of hypertension with antihypertensive medication. This is why it is vital to schedule consistent follow-ups with your primary care provider and engage in ongoing blood pressure monitoring.

As a separate aspect of addressing overall health, neuropsychological services can assist with improving the overall quality of life. This is discussed in more detail below.

Brain Protectant #4: Neuropsychological Services

The field of neuropsychology is dedicated to learning about and diagnosing conditions related to the brain and nervous system. The benefits of neuropsychological services can be summarized into three specific areas that can assist with warding off dementia-related conditions.

Benefit #1: Attaining an Accurate Diagnosis. A neuropsychological evaluation can help confirm or rule out a possible dementia condition.[45] Neuropsychological exams also complement or add clarity to neurological exams by a neurologist. The sooner a diagnosis is clarified, the sooner an appropriate treatment can be provided. For example, there are cognitive-enhancing medications that the U.S. Food and Drug Administration

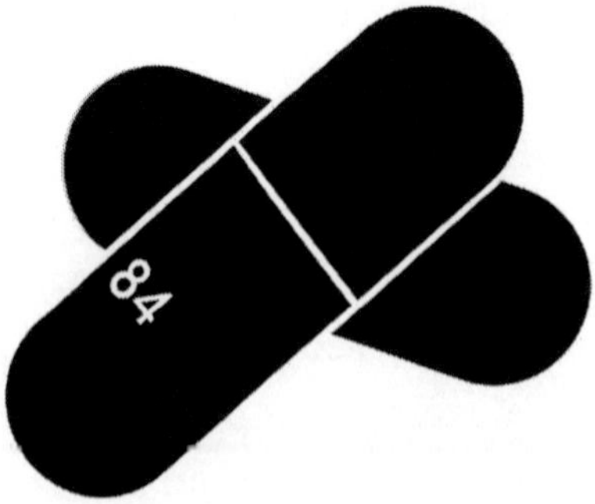

Benefits of Neuropsychological Services

Attaining an accurate diagnosis

Improving quality of life by making individual and treatment specific recommendations

Recieve an antidementia medication or supplement recommendation

(FDA) has approved for dementia conditions. These cognitive-enhancing medications are discussed later in this chapter.

Part of the reason it is essential to obtain early and accurate diagnosis of the presenting dementia condition is to tailor treatment specific to the dementia type. For example, in Lewy body dementia, the most appropriate pharmacological treatment is not with one of the known anti-dementia agents. Instead, patients with Lewy body dementia seem to respond best to levodopa (L-DOPA) therapy.[46,47]

Another reason to pursue healthcare exams is that potentially correctable causes of dementia may be detected. Sometimes referred to as "faux dementias," these conditions can return a person to baseline functioning once treated.

Vitamin B12 (cobalamin) deficiency is an example of a correctable cause of faux dementia.[48,49] Confirmation of B12 deficiency is usually done by a serum B12 level check pursued with a metabolic panel blood draw. B12 injections can reverse cognitive impairment, especially when the impairment is mild and of short duration.

Another example of reversible dementia is depression. As noted in previous chapters, depression can resemble dementia (sometimes referenced as pseudodementia). Neuropsychological exams can assist with differentiating between pseudodementia and a bona fide dementia condition. It is also essential to recognize that many features of patients with true dementia can be seen in psychiatric disorders. Psychiatric features may be an early symptom of subsequent cognitive decline.[50]

Before we move forward to the next benefit of the neuropsychological exam, an important point must be mentioned. I have been fortunate to assist with diagnosing and treating many elderly patients with hearing loss. I have also seen how cultural and linguistic factors associated with hearing loss can impede accurate diagnoses, preventing or delaying effective interventions that early treatment can bring. Hearing loss can present a litany of red herrings that can result in misdiagnosis. This is a point that can be elaborated further on another day. Still, it shows that choosing an appropriate provider may be just as important or more critical as receiving a workup.

Benefit #2: Developing an Individualized Treatment Plan. We can all agree that having an individualized treatment plan—specific to you—can lead to better health outcomes. This, in turn, can result in a higher quality of life. Individualized treatment plans can include specific recommendations for cognitive training to target areas of the brain to preserve cognitive functioning.

The research indicates that cognitive training has been found to improve cognitive and daily functioning for at least 5 years and up to 10 years.[51,52] Cognitive training has also been found to reduce the risk of dementia by 48%.[53] Engagement in cognitive training exercises at a clinic that provides these services tends to take about one hour. It can occur once weekly or daily, depending on your specific needs. These needs are usually determined based on the results of the neuropsychological exam.

One of the common questions patients frequently ask is whether doing a daily crossword puzzle, reading, or engaging in a card game can help ward off dementia. The answer is a resounding "Yes!" Generally speaking, the more the activity engages and stimulates the mind, the better it is as a mind exercise. Cognitive exercises are akin to physical exercise. As physical exercise is good for the heart, cognitive exercise is good for the head. Keeping your mind active, constantly learning new things, and being educated truly is a brain health intervention.

Of note is that receiving targeted cognitive training at a neuropsychological clinic can be better than simply engaging in daily cognitively stimulating activities. When working with a provider, you receive more than merely targeted training conducted by a professional. You also have access to routine follow-up care and monitoring of personal cognitive levels. Interactions with a provider can also provide a boost of self-esteem and confidence by providing reassurance that you are not alone in your progress towards improved cognitive functioning.[54]

Working with a provider also encourages diversity in cognitive training exercises to help you reap the most benefit in boosting brain health. Don't get me wrong—although a daily Sudoku puzzle is terrific for stimulating the brain, there can come the point of diminishing returns. As one becomes more adept at a given cognitive exercise, the more automated your brain becomes. The less mental willpower it takes to solve the problem. Just as a more vigorous effort with physical activity will reap more benefits than a "lighter" physical exercise regimen, the more novel and challenging a cognitive training exercise is, the better the benefit.[55]

Regarding stimulating cognitive training programs, the current best evidence points to games involving a dexterity component.[56-58] A great example of dexterity games are those video games requiring manual manipulation of controllers to move your avatar on the screen, thus fulfilling the dexterity component needed for maximum cognitive benefit.

***Benefit #3*: *Antidementia Medication or Supplement Recommendations*.** A thorough neuropsychological examination can provide guidance for medications or supplements that may benefit one's overall health. For instance, differentiating between anxiety, depression, and a dementia condition can be challenging to ascertain.[59,60] Clarifying a medical diagnosis allows for specific treatments that can include pharmacological workups as well as behavioral health recommendations.[61,62]

Before we get into the details of antidementia medications, it is essential to remember that no medicine has been shown to halt or reverse the progress of a dementia condition at this time.[63] At best, antidementia medications appear to result in a mild symptomatic improvement in cognitive functioning.[64] In a sense, they can "put lights on more often."

Unfortunately, the effect of antidementia medications tends to be transient—lasting only a few months.[65] After the antidementia drugs cease their effectiveness, the ordinary course of the dementia illness resumes.

Why are antidementia medications transient in nature? As we know, acetylcholine is an essential neurotransmitter for memory functions. Alzheimer's dementia is, after all, primarily driven by a loss of cholinergic neurons.[66] All but one of the antidementia drugs work by inhibiting the enzyme that breaks down acetylcholine. These medications are referenced as "acetylcholinesterase inhibitors." Inhibition of acetylcholine breakdown results in a natural increase of this neurotransmitter in the active synapse. As the dementia condition progresses, the efficacy of the antidementia drugs is lost because the brain stops producing acetylcholine.[67]

Several medication clinical trials are underway to address other aspects of dementia besides inhibiting acetylcholine breakdown.[68-71] These clinical trials aim to prevent the development of dementia—long before a slight decline in cognitive functioning or mild cognitive impairment manifests.[72] Addressing dementia at the preclinical stage requires avoiding the growth and accumulation of plaques in the gray matter areas of the brain.[73,74] Reducing or preventing the impaired clearance of beta-amyloid would hijack the cascade of negative effects that follow, such as hyperphosphorylation of tau protein and later formation of neurofibrillary tangles. A review of beta-amyloid's association with Alzheimer's is found in Chapter Two.

Currently Available Antidementia Medications (or Nootropics)

Let's talk about the antidementia medications we presently have that may assist with slowing down dementia symptoms. Antidementia medications are also sometimes referred to as nootropics. A nootropic is any substance that enhances cognition, memory, or learning. The first of these nootropics are the cholinesterase inhibitors.

Cholinesterase Inhibitors. The cholinesterase inhibitor medications include donepezil (brand name Aricept), rivastigmine (brand name Exelon), and galantamine (brand name Razadyne). Donepezil, rivastigmine, and galantamine are mainly effective in cases of mild to moderate dementia.

While the intended targets of the cholinesterase inhibitors are in the brain, these medications also increase levels of acetylcholine throughout the body.[75,76] The increase of acetylcholine throughout the body results in side effects associated with this neurotransmitter. These side effects include increased parasympathetic tone, including but not limited to nausea, diarrhea, gastrointestinal upset, and muscle cramps.

It is important to note that galantamine (Razadyne) has a "do not use" or "use with caution" warning for patients with renal (kidney) or hepatic (liver) impairment.[77] There is also a caution warning for patients who may have cardiac impairments.[78] For these reasons, galantamine should only be reserved for individuals who do not present with prior health conditions. Donepezil (Aricept) should also be used with caution in individuals who have cardiac impairment.[79]

NMDA Antagonist. Another type of antidementia agent—memantine (brand name Namenda)—is a medication that does not work as a cholinesterase inhibitor. Although memantine has a rather complicated neurotransmitter profile, it primarily works by mimicking and balancing the action of glutamate by blocking the flow through NMDA receptor channels.[80] Glutamate is a neurotransmitter that is thought to help with learning, memory, and clarity of thought processes.[81] However, too much glutamate stimulation leads to excitotoxicity, which results in loss of synaptic function and neuronal death.[82] Blockade of the flow of excess glutamate through the NMDA receptor channels allows better balance and preservation of cognitive functioning.

Of note, current evidence suggests that concomitant therapy with memantine and one of the cholinesterase inhibitors is significantly better than the use of one of the medications on its own.[83] The reason behind this is that none of the antidementia agents attacks the true pathophysiology of Alzheimer's (associated with neurofibrillary plaques and tangles in the brain that lead to neuronal cell death). It should also be noted that memantine is generally reserved for moderately severe cases of dementia (as opposed to a first-line treatment).[84]

Monoclonal Antibodies. An antidementia agent that received "accelerated approval" from the FDA in June of 2021 is aducanumab (brand name Aduhelm).[85] Like the other antidementia medications, aducanumab should only be used in early stages of Alzheimer's or mild cognitive impairment.

Aducanumab works as a monoclonal antibody engineered in a laboratory to stick to the amyloid protein that forms the plaques in the Alzheimer's brain.[86] Monoclonal antibodies are essentially artificial antibodies. Once the antibody has attached to the plaque, the body's immune system kicks in to remove the plaque, thinking it is a foreign invader. It is hoped that by removing the plaques, the brain cells will be protected from becoming tau tangles (which, as you may recall, kill the brain cells).[87] Retention of the brain cells can prevent the decline in memory and day-to-day functioning we would otherwise see in an untreated individual with Alzheimer's.

An aducanumab prescription requires a monthly intravenous infusion for as long as the individual takes the drug.[88] The reason for this is that aducanumab was noted in clinical trials to cause side effects of brain swelling. Intravenous infusions are required to monitor these potential side effects and know when to pause or stop the medication altogether. Approximately 30% of those receiving aducanumab were affected with brain swelling symptoms, with around 10% exhibiting tiny brain bleeds.[89,90] Although these side effects might be reversible, the risks are such that many practitioners may only use the medication in extreme cases.[91] Since aducanumab is a newer medication with "accelerated approval" from the FDA, the drug's effectiveness continues to be studied.

One antidementia drug, lecanemab, received FDA approval in January 2023. Lecanemab has a similar mechanism of action as aducanumab, working as a monoclonal antibody sticking to the amyloid protein that forms the plaques on the Alzheimer's brain.[92] While clinical trials have shown that lecanemab appears to slow the progression of cognitive decline by 27%, the findings are not, unfortunately, without some safety concerns. Akin to aducanumab, approximately 13% of trial participants receiving lecanemab experienced adverse events, such as brain swelling and bleeding.[93]

Psychostimulants. Psychostimulants are a final nootropic drug that is not necessarily an antidementia agent. One example of a psychostimulant that has been used in dementia research is modafinil (brand name Provigil).[94]

As a psychostimulant, modafinil improves alertness and focus. We know that improving alertness and focus is a key factor in cognitive performance.[95] The rationale is that by enhancing the ability to sustain concentration, we can stimulate the mind further, which can help slow dementia progression.

The actual data on the effectiveness of psychostimulants in slowing cognitive decline is mixed at best.[96] It also needs to be recognized that psychostimulants can sometimes result in the unwanted effect of exacerbating behavioral and psychological symptoms of dementia.

Future Possibility. Some evidence is beginning to arise that suggests that low doses of lithium may significantly delay the onset of dementia. The studies found that patients with mood disorders who took lithium had a lower incidence of dementia than similar patients who were not prescribed lithium.[97]

Prior lithium studies have found that communities with lithium concentrations in drinking water have lower suicide rates than the general population average.[98] These findings have prompted at least three investigations of lithium concentrations in drinking water and the incidence of dementia.[99-101] Of the three studies, two found a correlation supporting lithium's protective effects against dementia. The one negative study had average lithium exposures at unusually low levels.

Although we have some evidence suggesting an antidementia effect with low-dose lithium, more studies are needed to confirm these exciting findings. Further studies will help to ensure other evidence of lithium's antidementia protective effects and its safety for use. Fortunately, a study is underway that examines what appears to be lithium's promising antidementia potential.[102]

OTC Nootropic Supplements. Walk through the aisles of almost any vitamin or supplement store, and you will likely see at least one label or fold-up stand advertising the cognitive benefits of the supplement. Claims that the supplement will "enhance mental clarity," "improve memory," or "increase focus" abound. What do we make of all the hubbub? Since the promise of improved cognitive functioning appeals to everyone, it is no surprise that the market for such enhancements is enormous.

It is important to note that the FDA does not regulate the over-the-counter vitamin and supplement industry. This means that the FDA does not oversee product research, testing, or ingredient accuracy. The only issue the FDA may look into is supplements that make health claims related to treating specific diseases.[103] Thus, vitamin and supplement manufacturers can claim that their product helps with brain fog or memory loss. They cannot say that their supplement prevents or protects against dementia onset. Talk about how to get around the requirement to back up a claim that a given product is effective against specific neurodegenerative diseases!

Supplement manufacturers that claim to have conducted trials showing that their brand is effective must be viewed cautiously. When trials are paid for and overseen by the supplement manufacturers, this is a red flag and indicates biased results. For example, the inclusion criteria can be adjusted to reflect favorable outcomes to the supplement, and unfavorable results may be disregarded. Without the strict oversight that comes with FDA approval, it can be challenging to know what supplements are bona fide game changers in the cognitive enhancement arena. Especially in terms of brand supplements that claim to have proprietary and often unknown ingredients (sometimes referenced as a "proprietary nutritional blend").

That said, two specific minerals have at least some research regarding their potential to protect or enhance cognitive functioning: Coenzyme Q10 (CoQ10) and glutathione (sometimes referenced by the acronym GSH). As an antioxidant, CoQ10 assists with the health of neurons and brain functioning. CoQ10 serves as an energy source for the body's cells. Specifically, CoQ10 helps fuel adenosine triphosphate, or ATP, for mitochondria by converting fat and other substances into energy.[104] Since brain cells have a higher concentration of mitochondria than most other cells in the body, it is perhaps not surprising that CoQ10 has been known to lead to increased energy and enhanced cognition.

Animal studies have shown that CoQ10 is involved with anti-inflammation, vasoreactivity, and maintaining pH.[105] The evidence becomes murkier when considering whether CoQ10 has these same beneficial effects on the human brain.[106] While it is clear that low levels of CoQ10 in the body have been shown to bring on brain fog and general cognitive decline, what is less clear is whether CoQ10 supplements are effective in replacing these deficiencies.

Glutathione is another antioxidant that assists with the health of neurons and brain functioning. (Notice that antioxidant supplements are key here in their potentially protective effects on brain functioning.) Glutathione has been referenced as the "most important antioxidant" produced by cells in the body.[107] Within the mitochondria of cells, glutathione is thought to regulate apoptosis or neuronal cell death.

The problem with glutathione is its low bioavailability.[108] Bioavailability is the proportion of a drug or other substance that enters the body's circulation when introduced into the body and can have an active effect.[109] The precursor to glutathione, N-acetylcysteine, is another supplement that is sometimes used to increase glutathione production. Moreover, a prior study found that a sublingual administration of glutathione resulted in higher concentrations of oral glutathione or N-acetylcysteine.[110]

Research with other vitamins or minerals has produced results that might best be described as more of a "mixed bag." These other vitamins or minerals that have claimed protective effects against cognitive decline include omega-3 fatty acids (actual fish has proven benefits, not the supplement), ginkgo biloba, vitamin E, curcumin, and the B vitamins (B6, B12, and folic acid).[111]

No one-size-fits-all over-the-counter vitamin or mineral is a surefire means of protecting against cognitive decline. If this is true, why is there still a massive market for nootropics today? Part of the answer may be related to the fact that it is easier to take a pill than to implement the more surefire strategy of protecting against cognitive decline: lifestyle changes. Yes, the best way to incorporate supplements is by eating a healthy and well-balanced diet that includes nuts, fresh berries, healthy oils, and green, leafy vegetables (think Mediterranean diet). Regular physical exercise also supports healthy aging and brain functioning.

Brain Protectant #5: Maintaining or Developing Social Connections

Social connections matter for our cognitive health. Let's say that one more time. Social connections matter for our cognitive health. Although we've previously discussed the negative repercussions of loneliness and isolation on overall health and longevity, we cannot overstate the importance of developing and maintaining social connections as a vital brain-protectant step.

While some of us might fall on the introverted side of the spectrum, the need for at least some form of social connection is a deeply ingrained human characteristic. However, individuals on the introverted side of the spectrum may only need a little social interaction to feel content compared to someone who leans toward the extroverted side. What matters is the gap between the social interaction a person desires and how well they are getting these needs met."

Take, for example, being surrounded by people but still feeling lonely—a common scenario for individuals with hearing loss. Inaccessible communication can lead to feelings of isolation. As social creatures by nature, we humans need at least some meaningful connection with others, whether with one, a few, or many. Even though we are more "connected" today via social media apps (eg, Facebook, Twitter, Instagram), social connection is much more than this. Social connection is about connectedness or the extent to which we engage with essential people in our lives. This connectedness heightens our sense of belonging and well-being.

Don't get me wrong. Social media provides many benefits, especially for those of us with hearing loss, including background information we might have missed from casual in-person conversations. Social media updates can also provide fodder for later discussions with friends and family such as, "Congratulations on your newborn granddaughter!" or "Tell me more about your recent vacation!"

This is part of the reason that language deprivation or delay is a significant social justice issue within the deaf community. Well-meaning advocates of the vocal-auditory approach for deaf youth may not realize the long-term adverse effects that can result. Language barriers can lead to alienation from all communities. Such alienation is unnecessary and can be prevented. It takes a recognition of the need for reliable language access during the critical period of language development (birth to age five).

The natural inclination among those with late-onset hearing loss might be to pull away or withdraw from social engagements. Trying to engage with others when it is a struggle to comprehend communication can take time, energy, and, not to forget, courage. Developing and maintaining social connections in the face of late-onset hearing loss is vital.

Finding others with similar late-onset hearing loss experiences can help address difficulties associated with adjusting to a newfound hearing loss. Look for organizations online, such as the Hearing Loss Association of America (HLAA) or the Association of Late-Deafened Adults (ALDA). Local chapters of these organizations often have weekly or monthly meetings and activities to interact and learn from others experiencing similar circumstances.

One of the amazing things that our culturally Deaf community has that might be seen as an advantage over those with late-onset hearing loss is the generally solid social bonds found among individuals in this community. These strong social connections can aid resiliency against cognitive decline.

We also cannot forget the videophone technology that has been integral to our deaf community since the early 2000s. First introduced as an accommodation that allows our deaf community to connect with others who can hear via a sign language interpreter (or video relay service), the videophone provides a high-quality and secure means for deaf individuals to connect to one another.

Individuals with late-onset hearing loss may also use technology to interact with a friend or family member. Apps such as FaceTime, Zoom, or Google Meet allow an online video-to-video connection. There may also be a hidden advantage for the individual with late-onset hearing loss in using these apps: many provide voice-to-text captions of the communication. This feature can provide meaningful and impactful social interaction, which can be a boon for fostering social connections while removing other barriers, such as distance or time.

Key Takeaways

We've covered a lot of territory regarding protecting that precious noggin resting behind our eyes and between our ears. Overall, the tried-and-true protective measures we can take include:

- The "Scary E"—exercise. Exercise assists us with optimizing our cognitive functioning in a way unparalleled to supplements or prescription medications.
- Making small and simple changes in our nutrition routine can add up over time and improve overall brain health. The Mediterranean diet has the most evidence for preserving cognitive health.
- Monitoring blood pressure is key to knowing when to get needed treatment for hypertension or even hypotension.
- Obtaining a neuropsychological and neurological examination for an accurate diagnosis allows for developing a treatment plan tailored specifically to you, with recommendations for potentially needed antidementia medications.
- Social connections matter for our cognitive health. Maintaining or developing social connections is vital for aiding resilience against cognitive decline.

Recall that for someone in the early stages of cognitive decline, an antidementia medication such as rivastigmine or memantine can help allow for several more "good" months. When cognitive decline is more advanced, these medications may do little more than add to the side effect burden without improving clinically significant outcomes.

Can you believe it? We've come to the end of our journey together. The issue of hearing loss as it relates to cognition and dementia can fit into healthy aging in numerous ways. Persistence in learning, adapting, and implementing healthy lifestyle changes are vital in keeping cognitive decline at bay. The fact that you have picked up and read this book indicates that you are taking a step in the right direction, and I applaud your efforts.

It is important to remember that forgetfulness or repeating stories are not an indication that dementia looms on the horizon. Yes, it can be an early warning sign. But it does not always mean that cognitive functioning is doomed. We can still make changes and implement lifestyle adaptations to keep dementia at bay. Whether or not we have hearing loss, we have some control over where our mind goes as we age.

If there is one thing you take from this book, I hope it is the fact that it is never too late to start...anything. In our case, it is never too late to improve your lifestyle to maximize your chances of keeping dementia at bay. As George Bernard Shaw said, "You don't stop laughing when you grow old, you grow old when you stop laughing."

CHAPTER FIVE REFERENCES

1. Ratey JJ. *Spark: The Revolutionary New Science of Exercise and the Brain.* Little, Brown & Co; 2008.
2. Cotman CW, Berchtold NC, Christie L-A. Exercise builds brain health: key roles of growth factor cascades and inflammation. *Trends Neurosci.* 2007;30(9):464-472.
3. Alty J, Farrow M, Lawler K. Exercise and dementia prevention. *Pract Neurol.* 2020;20(3):234-240.
4. Chen F-T, Etnier JL, Chan K-H, Chiu P-K, Hung T-M, Chang Y-K. Effects of exercise training interventions on executive function in older adults: a systematic review and meta-analysis. *Sports Med.* 2020;50(8):1451-1467.
5. Hansen A. *The Real Happy Pill: Power Up Your Brain by Moving Your Body.* Simon & Schuster; 2017.
6. Nuzum H, Stickel A, Corona M, Zeller M, Melrose RJ, Wilkins SS. Potential benefits of physical activity in MCI and dementia. *Behav Neurol.* 2020.
7. Watt JA, Goodarzi Z, Veroniki AA, et al. Comparative efficacy of interventions for reducing symptoms of depression in people with dementia: systematic review and network meta-analysis. *BMJ.* 2021;372.
8. Naci H, Salcher-Konrad M, Dias S, et al. How does exercise treatment compare with antihypertensive medications? A network meta-analysis of 391 randomised controlled trials assessing exercise and medication effects on systolic blood pressure. *Br J Sports Med.* 2019;53(14):859-869.
9. Fiuza-Luces C, Garatachea N, Berger NA, Lucia A. Exercise is the real polypill. *Physiology.* 2013;28(5):330-358. doi: 10.1152/physiol.00019.2013
10. Northey JM, Cherbuin N, Pumpa KL, Smee DJ, Rattray B. Exercise interventions for cognitive function in adults older than 50: a systematic review with meta-analysis. *Br J Sports Med.* 2018;52(3):154-160.
11. Song D, Doris S, Li PW, Lei Y. The effectiveness of physical exercise on cognitive and psychological outcomes in individuals with mild cognitive impairment: a systematic review and meta-analysis. *Int J Nurs Stud.* 2018;79:155-164.

12. Zheng G, Xia R, Zhou W, Tao J, Chen L. Aerobic exercise ameliorates cognitive function in older adults with mild cognitive impairment: a systematic review and meta-analysis of randomised controlled trials. *Br J Sports Med.* 2016;50(23):1443-1450.
13. Rodrigues F, Teixeira DS, Neiva HP, Cid L, Monteiro D. Understanding exercise adherence: The predictability of past experience and motivational determinants. *Brain Sci.* 2020;10(2):98.
14. Saida TGRH, Sørensen TJ, Langberg H. Long-term exercise adherence after public health training in at-risk adults. *Ann Phys Rehabil Med.* 2017;60(4):237-243.
15. Kabat-Zinn J, Hanh TN. *Full Catastrophe Living: Using the Wisdom of Your Body and Mind to Face Stress, Pain, and Illness.* Delta; 2009.
16. Lopes S, Mesquita-Bastos J, Alves AJ, Ribeiro F. Exercise as a tool for hypertension and resistant hypertension management: current insights. *Integr Blood Press Control.* 2018;11:65.
17. Waheed S, Cannon CP. Cardiac rehabilitation reduces the long-term risk of death and cardiovascular complications. *Rev Cardiovasc Med.* 2010;11(3):181-185.
18. Agostinis-Sobrinho C, Ruiz JR, Moreira C, et al. Cardiorespiratory fitness and blood pressure: a longitudinal analysis. *J Pediatr.* 2018;192:130-135.
19. Dekleva M, Lazic JS, Arandjelovic A, Mazic S. Beneficial and harmful effects of exercise in hypertensive patients: the role of oxidative stress. *Hypertens Res.* 2017;40(1):15-20.
20. Lopes S, Félix G, Mesquita-Bastos J, Figueiredo D, Oliveira J, Ribeiro F. Determinants of exercise adherence and maintenance among patients with hypertension: a narrative review. *Rev Cardiovasc Med.* 2021;22(4):1271-1278.
21. Zotcheva E, Bergh S, Selbæk G, et al. Midlife physical activity, psychological distress, and dementia risk: the HUNT study. *J Alzheimers Dis.* 2018;66(2):825-833.
22. Kalback W, Esh C, Castaño EM, et al. Atherosclerosis, vascular amyloidosis and brain hypoperfusion in the pathogenesis of sporadic Alzheimer's disease. *Neurol Res.* 2004;26(5):525-539.

23. Shabir O, Berwick J, Francis SE. Neurovascular dysfunction in vascular dementia, Alzheimer's and atherosclerosis. *BMC Neurosci.* 2018;19(1):1-16.
24. O'Keefe JH, Gheewala NM, O'Keefe JO. Dietary strategies for improving post-prandial glucose, lipids, inflammation, and cardiovascular health. *J Am Coll Cardiol.* 2008;51(3):249-255.
25. Poznyak A, Grechko AV, Poggio P, Myasoedova VA, Alfieri V, Orekhov AN. The diabetes mellitus–atherosclerosis connection: the role of lipid and glucose metabolism and chronic inflammation. *Int J Mol Sci.* 2020;21(5):1835.
26. Firth J, Solmi M, Wootton RE, et al. A meta-review of "lifestyle psychiatry": the role of exercise, smoking, diet and sleep in the prevention and treatment of mental disorders. *World Psychiatry.* 2020;19(3):360-380.
27. Weaver CM. Diet, gut microbiome, and bone health. *Curr Osteoporo Rep.* 2015;13(2):125-130.
28. Guasch-Ferré M, Willett W. The Mediterranean diet and health: a comprehensive overview. *J Intern Med.* 2021;290(3):549-566.
29. Ramsey D. *Eat to Beat Depression and Anxiety: Nourish Your Way to Better Mental Health in Six Weeks.* HarperCollins; 2021.
30. Opie RS, O'Neil A, Jacka FN, Pizzinga J, Itsiopoulos C. A modified Mediterranean dietary intervention for adults with major depression: dietary protocol and feasibility data from the SMILES trial. *Nutr Neurosci.* 2018;21(7):487-501.
31. Guillaume C, De Alzaa F, Ravetti L. Evaluation of chemical and physical changes in different commercial oils during heating. *Acta Scientific Nutritional Health.* 2018;2(6):2-11.
32. Guo X, Park Y, Freedman ND, et al. Sweetened beverages, coffee, and tea and depression risk among older US adults. *PLoS One.* 2014;9(4):e94715. doi: 10.1371/journal.pone.0094715.
33. Magrone T, Russo MA, Jirillo E. Cocoa and dark chocolate polyphenols: from biology to clinical applications. *Front Immunol.* 2017:677.
34. Baranowski BJ, Marko DM, Fenech RK, Yang AJ, MacPherson RE. Healthy brain, healthy life: a review of diet and exercise interventions to promote brain health and reduce Alzheimer's disease risk. *Appl Physiol Nutr Metab.* 2020;45(10):1055-1065.

35. Jacka FN, Cherbuin N, Anstey KJ, Sachdev P, Butterworth P. Western diet is associated with a smaller hippocampus: a longitudinal investigation. *BMC Med.* 2015;13(1):1-8.
36. Debette S, Markus H. The clinical importance of white matter hyperintensities on brain magnetic resonance imaging: systematic review and meta-analysis. *BMJ.* 2010;341.
37. Yang Q, Chang A, Ritchey MD, Loustalot F. Antihypertensive medication adherence and risk of cardiovascular disease among older adults: a population-based cohort study. *J Am Heart Assoc.* 2017;6(6):e006056.
38. Fretheim A, Odgaard-Jensen J, Brørs O, et al. Comparative effectiveness of antihypertensive medication for primary prevention of cardiovascular disease: systematic review and multiple treatments meta-analysis. *BMC Med.* 2012;10(1):1-14.
39. Gronewold J, Jokisch M, Schramm S, et al. Association of blood pressure, its treatment, and treatment efficacy with volume of white matter hyperintensities in the population-based 1000BRAINS Study. *Hypertension.* 2021;78(5):1490-1501.
40. Wändell P, Carlsson AC, Sundquist J, Sundquist K. Antihypertensive drugs and relevant cardiovascular pharmacotherapies and the risk of incident dementia in patients with atrial fibrillation. *Int J Cardiol.* 2018;272:149-154.
41. Katzung BG, Trevor AJ. *Basic & Clinical Pharmacology.* McGraw-Hill; 2012.
42. Sawicka K, Szczyrek M, Jastrzebska I, Prasal M, Zwolak A, Daniluk J. Hypertension–the silent killer. *J Pre-Clin Clin Res.* 2011;5(2).
43. Kjeldsen SE. Hypertension and cardiovascular risk: general aspects. *Pharmacol Res.* 2018;129:95-99.
44. Mossello E, Pieraccioli M, Nesti N, et al. Effects of low blood pressure in cognitively impaired elderly patients treated with antihypertensive drugs. *JAMA Intern Med.* 2015;175(4):578-585.
45. Kawas C, Corrada M, Brookmeyer R, et al. Visual memory predicts Alzheimer's disease more than a decade before diagnosis. *Neurology.* 2003;60(7):1089-1093.
46. Molloy S, McKeith I, O'Brien J, Burn D. The role of levodopa in the management of dementia with Lewy bodies. *J Neurol*

Neurosurg Psychiatry. 2005;76(9):1200-1203.
47. Lucetti C, Logi C, Del Dotto P, et al. Levodopa response in dementia with Lewy bodies: a 1-year follow-up study. *Parkinsonism Relat Disord*. 2010;16(8):522-526.
48. Blundo C, Marin D, Ricci M. Vitamin B12 deficiency associated with symptoms of frontotemporal dementia. *Neurol Sci*. 2011;32(1):101-105.
49. Issac TG, Soundarya S, Christopher R, Chandra SR. Vitamin B12 deficiency: an important reversible co-morbidity in neuropsychiatric manifestations. *Indian J Psychol Med*. 2015;37(1):26-29.
50. Tripathi M, Vibha D. Reversible dementias. *Indian J Psychiatry*. 2009;51(Suppl1):S52.
51. Willis SL, Tennstedt SL, Marsiske M, et al. Long-term effects of cognitive training on everyday functional outcomes in older adults. *JAMA*. 2006;296(23):2805-2814.
52. Rebok GW, Ball K, Guey LT, et al. Ten-year effects of the ACTIVE cognitive training trial on cognition and everyday functioning in older adults. *J Am Geriatr Soc*. 2014;62(1):16.
53. Brain training reduces dementia risk across 10 years [press release]. American Psychological Association. August 4, 2016. Accessed November 3, 2022. https://www.apa.org/news/press/releases/2016/08/brain-training-dementia
54. Wampold BE. How important are the common factors in psychotherapy? An update. *World Psychiatry*. 2015;14(3):270-277.
55. Valenzuela MJ. Brain reserve and the prevention of dementia. *Curr Opin Psychiatry*. 2008;21(3):296-302.
56. Dove E, Astell AJ. The use of motion-based technology for people living with dementia or mild cognitive impairment: a literature review. *J Med Internet Res*. 2017;19(1):e6518.
57. Chao Y-Y, Scherer YK, Montgomery CA. Effects of using Nintendo Wii™ exergames in older adults: a review of the literature. *J Aging Health*. 2015;27(3):379-402.
58. Interview with Peter Whitehouse "How to Prevent Cognitive Decline." *The Carlat Psychiatry Podcast* with Chris Aiken and Kellie Newsome. December 13, 2021. https://www.

thecarlatreport.com/blogs/2-the-carlat-psychiatry-podcast/post/3592-how-to-prevent-cognitive-decline
59. Enache D, Winblad B, Aarsland D. Depression in dementia: epidemiology, mechanisms, and treatment. *Curr Opin Psychiatry*. 2011;24(6):461-472.
60. Muliyala KP, Varghese M. The complex relationship between depression and dementia. *Ann Indian Acad Neurol*. 2010;13(Suppl2):S69.
61. Downing LJ, Caprio TV, Lyness JM. Geriatric psychiatry review: differential diagnosis and treatment of the 3 D's-delirium, dementia, and depression. *Curr Psychiatry Rep*. 2013;15(6):1-10.
62. Herrmann N, Lanctôt KL, Hogan DB. Pharmacological recommendations for the symptomatic treatment of dementia: the Canadian Consensus Conference on the Diagnosis and Treatment of Dementia 2012. *Alzheimers Res Ther*. 2013;5(1):1-12.
63. Cui C-C, Sun Y, Wang X-Y, Zhang Y, Xing Y. The effect of anti-dementia drugs on Alzheimer disease-induced cognitive impairment: A network meta-analysis. *Medicine*. 2019;98(27).
64. Ihl R, Froelich L, Winblad B, et al. World Federation of Societies of Biological Psychiatry (WFSBP) guidelines for the biological treatment of Alzheimer's disease and other dementias. *World J Biol Psychiatry*. 2011;12(1):2-32.
65. VanDenBerg CM, Jann MW. Antidementia drugs. In: Jann MW, Penzak SR, Cohen LJ, eds. *Applied Clinical Pharmacokinetics and Pharmacodynamics of Psychopharmacological Agents*. Springer; 2016: 329-349. doi: 10.1007/978-3-319-27883-4
66. Ferreira-Vieira TH, Guimaraes IM, Silva FR, Ribeiro FM. Alzheimer's disease: targeting the cholinergic system. *Curr Neuropharmacol*. 2016;14(1):101-115.
67. Clarke NA, Francis PT. Cholinergic and glutamatergic drugs in Alzheimer's disease therapy. *Expert Rev Neurother*. 2005;5(5):671-682.
68. Joseph-Mathurin N, Llibre-Guerra JJ, Li Y, et al. Amyloid-related imaging abnormalities in the DIAN-TU-001 Trial of Gantenerumab and Solanezumab: lessons from a trial

in dominantly inherited Alzheimer disease. *Ann Neurol.* 2022;92(5):729-744.

69. Aisen P, Bateman R, Carrillo M, et al. Platform trials to expedite drug development in Alzheimer's disease: a report from the EU/US CTAD Task Force. *J Prev Alzheimers Dis.* 2021;8(3):306-312.
70. Ngolab J, Donohue M, Belsha A, et al. Feasibility study for detection of retinal amyloid in clinical trials: The Anti-Amyloid Treatment in Asymptomatic Alzheimer's Disease (A4) trial. *Alzheimers Dement (Amst).* 2021;13(1):e12199.
71. Rygiel K. Novel strategies for Alzheimer's disease treatment: An overview of anti-amyloid beta monoclonal antibodies. *Indian J Pharmacol.* 2016;48(6):629.
72. Wisniewski T, Konietzko U. Amyloid-β immunisation for Alzheimer's disease. *Lancet Neurol.* 2008;7(9):805-811.
73. Prasansuklab A, Tencomnao T. Amyloidosis in Alzheimer's disease: the toxicity of amyloid beta (Aβ), mechanisms of its accumulation and implications of medicinal plants for therapy. *Evid Based Complement Alternat Med.* 2013;2013.
74. Lozupone M, Solfrizzi V, D'Urso F, et al. Anti-amyloid-β protein agents for the treatment of Alzheimer's disease: an update on emerging drugs. *Expert Opin Emerg Drugs.* 2020;25(3):319-335.
75. Wilkinson DG, Francis PT, Schwam E, Payne-Parrish J. Cholinesterase inhibitors used in the treatment of Alzheimer's disease. *Drugs Aging.* 2004;21(7):453-478.
76. Singh R, Sadiq NM. Cholinesterase inhibitors. StatPearls [Internet]. Updated February 25, 2023. Accessed December 5, 2022. https://www.ncbi.nlm.nih.gov/books/NBK544336/
77. Zhao Q, Iyer GR, Verhaeghe T, Truyen L. Pharmacokinetics and safety of galantamine in subjects with hepatic impairment and healthy volunteers. *J Clin Pharmacol.* 2002;42(4):428-436.
78. Committee ADRA. Deaths with galantamine in mild cognitive impairment studies. *Australian Adverse Drug Reactions Bulletin.* 2006;25(1):2.
79. Sato K, Urbano R, Yu C, et al. The effect of donepezil treatment on cardiovascular mortality. *Clin Pharmacol Ther.* 2010;88(3):335-338.

80. Danysz W, Parsons CG, Möbius H-J, Stöffler A, Quack G. Neuroprotective and symptomatological action of memantine relevant for Alzheimer's disease—a unified glutamatergic hypothesis on the mechanism of action. *Neurotox Res.* 2000;2(2):85-97.
81. McEntee WJ, Crook TH. Glutamate: its role in learning, memory, and the aging brain. *Psychopharmacology.* 1993;111(4):391-401.
82. Svob D, Konjevod M, Sagud M, et al. Personalizing the care and treatment of Alzheimer's disease: an overview. *Pharmgenomics Pers Med.* 2021 May;14:631-653. doi: 10.2147/PGPM.S284615.
83. Herrmann N, Li A, Lanctôt K. Memantine in dementia: a review of the current evidence. *Expert Opin Pharmacother.* 2011;12(5):787-800.
84. McShane R, Westby MJ, Roberts E, et al. Memantine for dementia. *Cochrane Database Syst Rev.* 2019(3).
85. Steinbrook R. The accelerated approval of aducanumab for treatment of patients with Alzheimer disease. *JAMA Intern Med.* 2021;181(10):1281-1281.
86. Sevigny J, Chiao P, Bussière T, et al. The antibody aducanumab reduces Aβ plaques in Alzheimer's disease. *Nature.* 2016;537(7618):50-56.
87. A new Alzheimer's drug has been approved. But should you take it? Harvard Health Publishing. July 15, 2021. Accessed December 28, 2022. https://www.health.harvard.edu/blog/a-new-alzheimers-drug-has-been-approved-but-should-you-take-it-202106082483
88. Padda IS, Parmar M. Aducanumab. StatPearls [Internet]. Updated January 17, 2023. Accessed December 29, 2022. https://www.ncbi.nlm.nih.gov/books/NBK573062/
89. Watson LC, Juman R. AMDA position statement on aducanumab. *J Am Med Dir Assoc.* 2021;22(9):1777.
90. Schulman KA, Greicius MD, Richman B. Will CMS find aducanumab reasonable and necessary for Alzheimer disease after FDA approval? *JAMA.* 2021;326(5):383-384.
91. VandeVrede L, Gibbs DM, Koestler M, et al. Symptomatic amyloid-related imaging abnormalities in an APOE ε4/ε4

patient treated with aducanumab. *Alzheimers Dement (Amst).* 2020;12(1):e12101.

92. Shi M, Chu F, Zhu F, Zhu J. Impact of anti-amyloid-β monoclonal antibodies on the pathology and clinical profile of Alzheimer's disease: a focus on aducanumab and lecanemab. *Front Aging Neurosci.* 2022;14.
93. van Dyck CH, Swanson CJ, Aisen P, et al. Lecanemab in early Alzheimer's disease. *New Engl J Med.* 2022.
94. Ballon JS, Feifel D. A systematic review of modafinil: potential clinical uses and mechanisms of action. *J Clin Psychiatry.* 2006;67(4):554-566.
95. Turner DC, Robbins TW, Clark L, Aron AR, Dowson J, Sahakian BJ. Cognitive enhancing effects of modafinil in healthy volunteers. *Psychopharmacology.* 2003;165(3):260-269.
96. Dolder CR, Nicole Davis L, McKinsey J. Use of psychostimulants in patients with dementia. *Ann Pharmacother.* 2010;44(10):1624-1632.
97. Ishii N, Terao T, Hirakawa H. The present state of lithium for the prevention of dementia related to Alzheimer's dementia in clinical and epidemiological studies: a critical review. *Int J Environ Res Public Health.* 2021;18(15):7756.
98. Barjasteh-Askari F, Davoudi M, Amini H, et al. Relationship between suicide mortality and lithium in drinking water: a systematic review and meta-analysis. *J Affect Disord.* 2020;264:234-241.
99. Kessing LV, Gerds TA, Knudsen NN, et al. Association of lithium in drinking water with the incidence of dementia. *JAMA Psychiatry.* 2017;74(10):1005-1010.
100. McGrath JJ, Berk M. Could lithium in drinking water reduce the incidence of dementia? *JAMA Psychiatry.* 2017;74(10):983-984.
101. Fajardo VA, Fajardo VA, LeBlanc PJ, MacPherson RE. Examining the relationship between trace lithium in drinking water and the rising rates of age-adjusted Alzheimer's disease mortality in Texas. *J Alzheimers Dis.* 2018;61(1):425-434.
102. Hampel H, Lista S, Mango D, et al. Lithium as a treatment for Alzheimer's disease: the systems pharmacology perspective. *J Alzheimers Dis.* 2019;69(3):615-629.

103. Marcus DM. Dietary supplements: What's in a name? What's in the bottle? *Drug Test Anal.* 2016;8(3-4):410-412.
104. Forester BP, Harper DG, Georgakas J, Ravichandran C, Madurai N, Cohen BM. Antidepressant effects of open label treatment with coenzyme Q10 in geriatric bipolar depression. *J Clin Psychopharmacol.* 2015;35(3):338.
105. Yang X, Dai G, Li G, Yang ES. Coenzyme Q10 reduces β-amyloid plaque in an APP/PS1 transgenic mouse model of Alzheimer's disease. *J Mol Neurosci.* 2010;41(1):110-113.
106. Ferrante RJ, Andreassen OA, Dedeoglu A, et al. Therapeutic effects of coenzyme Q10 and remacemide in transgenic mouse models of Huntington's disease. *J Neurosci.* 2002;22(5):1592-1599.
107. Forman HJ, Zhang H, Rinna A. Glutathione: overview of its protective roles, measurement, and biosynthesis. *Mol Aspects Med.* 2009;30(1-2):1-12.
108. Dringen R. Metabolism and functions of glutathione in brain. *Prog Neurobiol.* 2000;62(6):649-671.
109. Price G, Patel DA. Drug bioavailability. StatPearls [Internet]. Updated June 23, 2022. Accessed January 3, 2023. https://www.ncbi.nlm.nih.gov/books/NBK557852/
110. Schmitt B, Vicenzi M, Garrel C, Denis FM. Effects of N-acetylcysteine, oral glutathione (GSH) and a novel sublingual form of GSH on oxidative stress markers: a comparative crossover study. *Redox Biology.* 2015;6:198-205.
111. Dangour AD, Whitehouse PJ, Rafferty K, et al. B-vitamins and fatty acids in the prevention and treatment of Alzheimer's disease and dementia: a systematic review. *J Alzheimers Dis.* 2010;22(1):205-224.

ABOUT THE AUTHOR

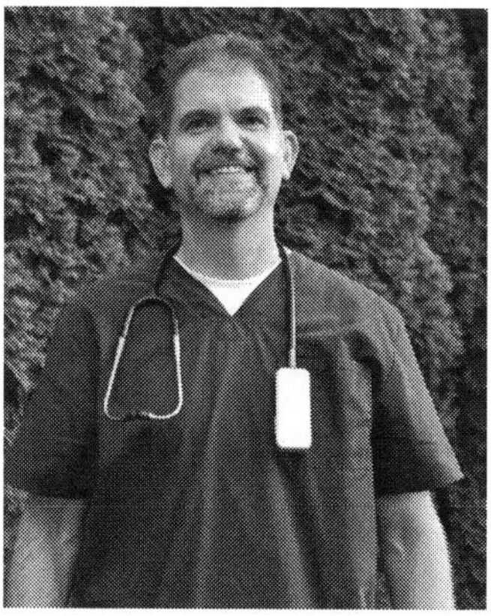

Dr. Jaime Wilson, Ph.D., ABN, ABPP, is a prescribing medical psychologist and board-certified neuropsychologist in full-time private practice both in Washington and in the nation. He holds privileges at several area hospitals and has worked extensively with physicians, other healthcare providers, and forensic experts, providing neuropsychological evaluations across the United States. The field of neuropsychology is dedicated to learning about and diagnosing conditions related to the brain and nervous system.

Dr. Wilson has served as president of the Association of Medical Professionals with Hearing Losses, serves on the Diversity Council for the Society of Prescribing Psychology, and chairs the American Board of Professional Neuropsychology Diversity Committee.

Born deaf, Dr. Wilson grew up wearing bilateral hearing aids and primarily communicated using spoken language. Today, in addition to spoken language, he also uses American Sign Language. He resides in Olympia, Washington, with his wife, also deaf and a registered nurse, their three kids, and a King Charles Spaniel named Pepper Jack.

To have Dr. Wilson speak at your next event, visit www.wilsonclinical.com/resources/#presentations.

ONLINE RESOURCES

- Dr. Wilson discusses cognitive decline and hearing loss on "Deaf Health Talk" hosted by the University of Michigan Medicine: https://www.youtube.com/watch?v=r7A0SXt-6Bo.
- Dr. Wilson provides a video podcast for Docs with Disabilities: https://podcasts.apple.com/us/podcast/docs-with-disabilities/id1474844514

Made in the USA
Monee, IL
25 August 2023

41604534R00087